Yoga for Healthy Lower Backs

Alison Trewhela Iyengar Yoga Assoc. (UK)
Anna Semlyen British Wheel of Yoga

Lotus Publishing
Chichester, England

Published in 2011 by **Lotus Publishing**, Apple Tree Cottage, Inlands Road, Nutbourne, Chichester, PO18 8RJ, UK.

Disclaimer

The content of this book is believed to be correct at the time of printing, but does not constitute specific advice for any particular reader's situation. Readers should seek expert or professional advice if in doubt about whether any of the recommendations would be appropriate for themselves. In any case, we advise that you ask your GP before attempting to follow the yoga presented in this manual and strongly advise you to also seek out the guidance of a fully-qualified yoga teacher.

Photo Acknowledgements

With Thanks to theStudent Models From Alison Trewhela's Iyengar. Yoga Classes At theAmazing Eco-Venue of theZedshed, Jubilee Wharf, Commercial Road, Penryn, Cornwall.

Cover Design Wendy Craig, Esme Lyall and Alison Trewhela
Text Design Wendy Craig
Photographs Alan and Alison Trewhela
Yoga Artwork Perran Trewhela, www.perrantrewhela.com
Printed and Bound in the UK by Scotprint

British Library Cataloguing-in-Publication Data
A CIP record for this book is available from the British Library
ISBN 978 1 905367 27 6

Contents

About This Book

As used alongside a three month course

This manual was first written by Alison Trewhela and Anna Semlyen for participants on a Randomised Controlled Trial of Yoga for Chronic Low Back Pain, conducted by **The University of York's York Trials Unit**, **The Department of Health Sciences**, and sponsored by **The University of York**, UK.

This research trial was generously funded by *Arthritis Research UK*.

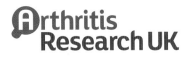

Providing answers today and tomorrow

The yoga in this manual was compiled by Alison Trewhela, *Iyengar Yoga Association (UK)* with contributions from Anna Semlyen, *British Wheel of Yoga*.

The *Iyengar Yoga Association (UK)* and the *British Wheel of Yoga* have been supportive of this research trial and the yoga programme from the outset and believe in its value.

The trial's yoga classes were taught, using this manual, by IYA(UK) and British Wheel of Yoga teachers specifically trained by Alison Trewhela in how to deliver this yoga programme to newcomers to yoga with low back pain. A proportion of the royalties from this book will contribute towards further research (going to Arthritis Research UK and also to The University of York).

For more information

www.yogaforbacks.co.uk, the *Yoga for Healthy Lower Backs* website, which includes how to find a trained teacher, the *Yoga for Healthy Lower Backs* Relaxations CD, and more.

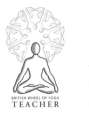

BRITISH WHEEL OF YOGA
TEACHER

IYENGAR YOGA
ASSOCIATION
OF THE UNITED KINGDOM

www.yogatrewhela.co.uk – Alison Trewhela's yoga site
www.yogainyork.co.uk – Anna Semlyen's yoga site
www.yogatrial.co.uk – The University of York research site for the trial

Revised Yoga for Healthy Lower Backs – Students' Manual

This manual was originally written for volunteers with low back problems, who had already seen their GP. Their doctor's practice sent them a letter inviting them to apply to take part in research called a *pragmatic multi-centred randomised controlled trial of yoga for chronic low back pain.*

In the trial, this manual was given to chronic (long-lasting) low back pain sufferers on arrival at their first specialist yoga class. A block of 12 weekly classes were taught to these beginning yoga students by highly-experienced, qualified and insured teachers from either the British Wheel of Yoga or Iyengar Yoga Association (UK). Teachers had invested their time in additional training in, and personal practice of, the *Yoga for Healthy Lower Backs* programme devised especially for this trial.

To gain the maximum benefit from this manual and to learn how to do yoga for your back safely and correctly, you are strongly advised to seek out a trained teacher via the *www.yogaforbacks.co.uk* website.

Various people were not allowed to become yoga students on the trial, including:

- Pregnant women (who require many modifications to yoga)
- Those who had previously had spinal surgery
- Anyone who could not get up off the floor unaided
- Those who could not walk up and down stairs
- People with any of the symptoms or a diagnosis of serious spinal disease or pathology (Also See Section 13).
- Anyone not experiencing back pain at the outset of the trial or scoring under 4 on the Roland-Morris Disability Questionnaire, (although the authors believe there is already some evidence that this programme will act preventatively)
- Those who had practised yoga at a class twice a month or more in the last 6 months (in order that the trial yoga classes could show a benefit)
- People who had been involved in another trial for their back pain in the past 6 months

- People under 18 and over 65 years of age (as it is more difficult to get research approval for studies with children and because older people are more likely to have other conditions as well as back pain that may require extra modifications of the yoga)
- People with a history of drug, alcohol or mental health issues as judged by their GP (due to unreliability of answers)
- Potential trial participants' GPs were asked whether there was any reason (back-related or otherwise) that they should not take part in the yoga.

Bearing the above in mind, we strongly advise you to seek the advice of your GP if you are at all concerned about whether to start to practise yoga.

In the trial, the yoga poses and relaxation techniques were practised at home within the practice sequences (CORE A, etc.). The poses were gradually taught and introduced to students in a carefully-designed, specialised, series of 12 differing yoga classes. These had an average of 10 participants and a maximum of 15. Classes lasted for 75 minutes and were themed to focus on yogic philosophical topics such as 'Comfort' or 'Strength'.

Although the general public will buy this book, we advise them to seek out a qualified yoga teacher via the www.yogaforbacks.co.uk website. They could ask their own local yoga teacher to attend one of our *Yoga for Healthy Lower Backs* training courses and that the yoga teacher will then become fully qualified and gain a depth of knowledge of the yoga poses contained within the sequences, along with a thorough understanding of how to tailor the yoga to individual needs.

As well as this manual, yoga participants were given the *Yoga for Healthy Lower Backs* Relaxations CD and a yoga mat to encourage home practice, plus a copy of *The Back Book* (a short educational booklet published by TSO).

If you are a yoga teacher and are interested in finding out how to train in this yoga programme, please refer to 15 'Four Day Training Course'.

For a full description of the trial's research methodology and results, visit *www.yogatrial.co.uk* and *www.annals.org*.

Acknowledgements

Trial Management Committee

Professor David J. Torgerson, Principal Investigator and Director of York Trials Unit, Department of Health Sciences, The University of York

Alison Trewhela, Iyengar Yoga Practitioner, Cornwall and Switzerland

Anna Semlyen, BWY Yoga Practitioner, York

Professor John D. Aplin, Professor of Reproductive Biomedicine and Iyengar Yoga Practitioner, University of Manchester

Helen E. Tilbrook, Research Fellow and Trial Co-ordinator, York Trials Unit, The University of York

Helen Cox, Research Fellow and Trial Co-ordinator, York Trials Unit, The University of York

Professor Ian Watt, Professor of Primary & Community Care, The University of York

Professor Jennifer Klaber-Moffett, Physiotherapist & Professor of Rehabilitation, formerly at the Institute for Rehabilitation, University of Hull and co-author of *The Back Book* and other back pain books.

Ben Cross, Catherine E. Hewitt, Shalmini Jayakody and Arthur Kang'ombe, Statisticians, York Trials Unit

Ling-Hsiang Chuang and Marta Soares, Health Economists, York Trials Unit

Other Staff at The University of York

Dominic Ennis, Multimedia Producer, who recorded and mastered the trial's *Yoga for Healthy Lower Backs* Relaxations CD

Secretarial and Business support staff at York Trials Unit, Intellectual Property Rights and Publicity Departments

Independent Trial Steering Committee

Professor Ian Roberts, Professor of Epidemiology, London School of Hygiene & Tropical Medicine

Dr. Tony Johnson, MRC Biostatistics Unit, Institute of Public Health, Cambridge

Dr. Isabelle Boutron, MD, Département d'Epidémiologie, Biostatistique et Recherche Clinique, Groupe Hospitalier Bichat-Claude Bernard, Paris

Dr. Lisa Roberts, Lecturer and Superintendent Physiotherapist, University of Southampton

Special Thanks To

- Arthritis Research UK for funding this research

- The back pain sufferers who took part in the research and filled in questionnaires

- The many yoga teachers who have been consulted and helped with producing the yoga contained within this manual

- IYA (UK) and BWY

- The dedicated 20 yoga teachers who trained for the trial, 12 of whom taught the trial's classes

- The models whose photographs are used in this manual and the venue, The ZedShed, Jubilee Wharf, Penryn, Cornwall

- The NHS Primary Care Trusts and GP Practises who contributed to the research by sending letters to patients asking them to volunteer for the trial in York, Cornwall, Manchester and London

- Roland-Morris Disability Questionnaire authors Prof. Martin O. Roland and R. W. Morris

- Lotus Publishing

- Esme Lyall for her help with the book colours and covers

- Yogacharya Sri B.K.S. Iyengar for his inspiration and lifelong dedication to spreading knowledge of yoga

- Perran Trewhela for his inspirational yoga artwork www.perrantrewhela.com

Introduction

Yoga is an excellent research-proven method for improving your back health. This book is most usefully used as a guide and adjunct to a *Yoga for Healthy Lower Backs* course, which comprises of 12 completely differentiated, weekly, 75-minute classes. Its main aim is to enable people attending classes to practice yoga postures and relaxation at home. Instructions and photographs are provided.

You may find the first half of this book the most useful. Expect to refer frequently to the practice sequences and practice diaries. The practice sequences give a name, a photograph and the order and number of repetitions of each yoga pose.

If you are attending a *Yoga for Healthy Lower Backs* course, Chapter 10, the longest section, is mainly for reference and further studies – although teachers will find it essential reading. Refer to it if you have any doubts about particular yoga poses or would like alternatives. It gives detailed instructions and is designed to help you understand how each individual yoga pose benefits your body, your mind and your whole being.

This book includes:

- Pain Relief Poses for when you have a painful back (7: 'What to Do If You Get a Sign of a Painful Back Episode'),
- A CORE yoga programme and a PROGRESSIVE programme of yoga poses (8: 'Yoga Sequences').
- Practising the CORE poses regularly and correctly will be enough to improve, and then maintain, your back health.
- The PROGRESSIVE poses are for when you feel that you can easily and comfortably do the CORE poses and for when you want a change. They can act as a bridge towards joining a general yoga class and/or can enable you to regain more flexibility, strength and confidence in your back when wishing to return to activities such as sport or gardening.

We strongly recommend that students practise yoga at home as well as go to a yoga class. The authors believe attending classes will, in itself, promote improved well-being. Home practice will help you to retain and build on the benefits to your strength, mobility and relaxation. Practising by yourself will mean that you can feel better all week, not just on the day of the class or the day after.

The yoga teachers who have completed the *Yoga for Healthy Lower Backs* training are experienced. They have mainly qualified with either the British Wheel of Yoga or Iyengar Yoga Association (UK) organisations and have completed additional training in yoga for the health of the lower back. Details of these yoga organisations are in 14 and qualified teacher lists are at *www. yogaforbacks.co.uk.*

Please consult a yoga teacher for clarification if you are unsure of anything.

We do not recommend that this programme is followed by pregnant women, as it requires considerable adaptation to make it appropriate.

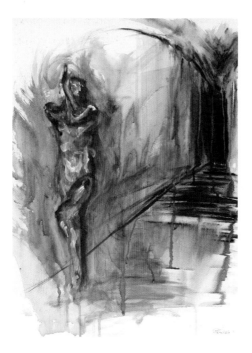

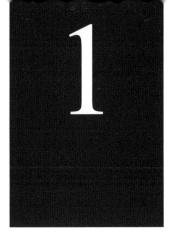

1   What is Yoga?

Choosing to learn and practise yoga is a positive step to helping the health of your back. The Sanskrit word '*Yoga*' refers to union between the body, breath, mind and the emotions. Yoga is a system of knowledge about well-being that comes from India and is thousands of years old. It is not a religion.

Physical postures, or poses, are the best known aspects of yoga. They promote strength, flexibility and good health so that we look and feel better. Our bodies need to be used regularly: a sedentary lifestyle, with its limited range of mostly repetitive daily movements, does not give the stretching, strengthening and relaxing that we need. Regular practice of yoga postures will raise self-awareness and physical and mental health. Yoga aims to enable people to enjoy a comfortable, steady posture with an alert mind. Learning to relax, attend to the breath and mental focus are therefore important aspects of yoga.

- Therapeutic yoga can be done to alleviate problems and also for prevention

- Yoga is often taught in classes. It can also be learnt one-to-one with a teacher

- As was offered in our yoga trial, we recommend that you attend regular weekly lessons with a qualified *Yoga for Healthy Lower Backs* teacher. As yoga is a movement skill, it will take longer to learn alone from books, DVDs or videos

- Once you have learnt how to practise yoga in a class, it is recommended that exercises are also done at home. The full benefits of yoga are more likely with regular, disciplined and persistent home practice

- Aim to keep a positive attitude and remind yourself that you do want to improve

▪ Stress and emotional factors contribute to back problems. Aim to reduce persistent high levels of stress in your life

▪ Do not expect improvement in your back pain overnight. But do feel your body accepting and enjoying its new flexibility, strength, relaxation, alignment and postural balance

▪ Do expect to feel better. Yoga can give a sense of well-being that will affect not only your back but other parts of your body, your mind, breathing, emotions and your life

We feel sure that you will enjoy learning yoga and will continue learning and practising it into the future.

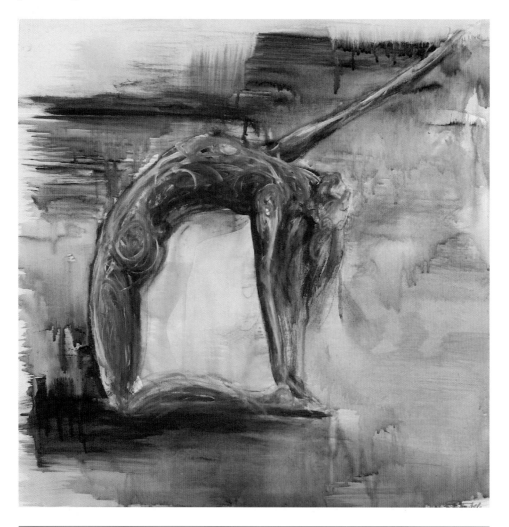

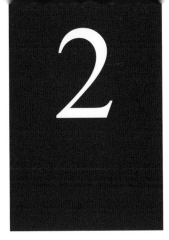

2

Results from the *Yoga for Healthy Lower Backs* Trial and Other Related Research

This Students' Manual was designed as a complementary educational aid to be used along with yoga classes taught to participants in research based at The University of York, Department of Health Sciences, York Trials Unit, UK. Trial results were published in a US medical journal in November 2011 (*Annals of Internal Medicine*, 'Yoga for chronic low back pain: a randomized trial'). This trial, one of the largest yoga trials worldwide, aimed to determine the effectiveness and cost-effectiveness of yoga designed for people who had seen their GP about chronic low back pain. Effects were rigorously compared with a control group receiving usual care and studied 313 participants.

Some of the main interpretations of the trial are (Tilbrook, et al. 2011):

'Conclusion: Offering a twelve-week yoga program of yoga to adults with chronic or recurrent low back pain led to greater improvements in back function than usual care.'

'Yoga appears to be a safe and effective activity that clinicians could consider recommending for patients with a history of low back pain.'

'The program was acceptable to, and taught by teachers from two yoga associations.'

'...the yoga group had higher pain self-efficacy scores at 3 and 6 months'

'Results: The yoga group had better back function at 3, 6 and 12 months than the usual care group.'

'The adjusted mean RMDQ score was 2.17 points (95% CI; 1.03 to 3.31 points) lower in the yoga group at 3 months, 1.48 points (CI 0.33 to 2.62 points) lower at 6 months and 1.57 points (CI 0.42 to 2.71 points)'.

12 experienced yoga teachers taught the 12-class 'Yoga for Healthy Lower Backs' course. 20 teachers were trained in the programme to allow for cover and quality control. Most previous trials had only used one teacher; a strength of this trial was that it aimed to ensure that it was not just one skilled teacher who could obtain an effect. It used teachers from the two most prominent

yoga organisations in the UK – The British Wheel of Yoga and Iyengar Yoga Association (UK). Yoga was taught in five locations (Cornwall, Manchester, North London, West London and York). Classes had an average allocation of approx. 10 students, with a maximum of 15. The statistical methods used to judge how much improvement stemmed from offering yoga allowed for possible confounding factors, including location, age, gender and duration of back pain.

The trial's yoga experts believed that those who practised at least twice a week would gain the most long-term benefit, so participants were encouraged to practise yoga at home. Over half (76 out of the 126 who answered the question) of those attending the 'Yoga for Healthy Lower Backs' course were continuing to practise yoga at home 9 months after the end of their yoga course. The most common frequency of yoga practice was twice a week for the yoga group.

The main outcome measure was the Roland-Morris Disability Questionnaire (RMDQ) score. This is a self-administered measure in which greater levels of disability are reflected by higher numbers on a 24-point scale. The RMDQ was measured at the start of the trial and at 3, 6, and 12 months. The '3 month time-point' corresponded to the end of the series of 12 (one per week), 75-minute yoga classes. The 313 trial participants were divided into the 'yoga group' (156 people) and the control or 'usual care group' (157) and compared.

Yoga was associated with a statistically and clinically significant improvement (compared to the non-yoga group) at 3 months on the RMDQ (2.17 points) and a significant difference in favour of yoga (1.57 points) was maintained 12 months after the beginning of the trial, even though the yoga classes had finished 9 months previously. At 3 months the participants who received yoga could on average do an extra two additional activities as shown on the RMDQ questionnaire compared to those who received usual care.

Improvements in Confidence in Being Able to Look After Oneself: This trial also showed positive results for yoga participants (compared to the usual care group at 3 and 6 months) according to a Pain Self-Efficacy Questionnaire.

For full references to published papers from this trial please refer to links on *www.yogatrial.co.uk* (University of York) or *www.yogaforbacks.co.uk*.

RMDQ Scores Over Time – Usual Care Group versus Yoga Group

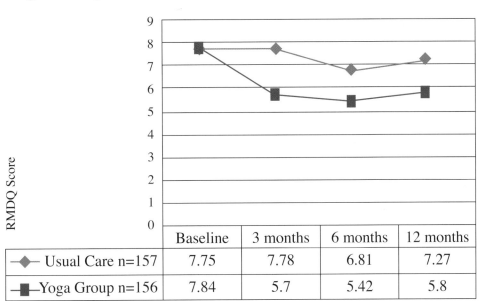

	Baseline	3 months	6 months	12 months
—◆— Usual Care n=157	7.75	7.78	6.81	7.27
—■—Yoga Group n=156	7.84	5.7	5.42	5.8

Comparison With Other Back Care Trials Using the RMDQ

The UK BEAM trial (2004) on manipulation for back pain at 3 months, showed a beneficial difference of 1.57 RMDQ points, whilst group exercise taught by physiotherapists gave a difference of 1.36 points, and manipulation plus exercise gave a difference of 1.87 points. At 12 months, manipulation showed a 1.01 point difference with exercise classes showing a 0.39 point difference.

6 sessions of group Cognitive Behavioural Therapy gave a difference of 1.10 points at 3 months compared to usual care.

A trial of the Alexander technique showed at 3 months that 6 x 'one-to-one' individual sessions gave a 1.71 difference, and 24 x 'one-to-one' individual sessions gave a 2.91 difference.

Consequently, referral to yoga (2.17 points at 3 months and 1.37 at 12 months) seems to be at the higher end of rigorously researched treatment interventions that have been shown to be effective.

Other Back Pain Exercise Research

The Back Book (2002), written by a team of health experts, concludes that the best way to deal with back pain is to "get back active". The back is designed for movement and needs a lot of it. "The sooner you get moving and doing your ordinary activities the sooner you will feel better."

So what kind of activity is best?   Standard exercise treatments, though widely used have had only a small effect on back pain (UK BEAM, 2004). Manipulation treatments, with a physiotherapist, chiropractor or osteopath are better than exercise alone, but are costly and are not widely available on the NHS (UK BEAM, 2004).

Yoga offers both physical exercise and mental focus. This makes it a very suitable therapy for low back pain. Partly as a result of numerous American studies, yoga is recommended in US back care guidance.

A randomised controlled trial in the USA has shown that low back patients who attended yoga classes had significantly less pain after 14 weeks compared with those in an exercise control group (Sherman et al, 2005). The improvement at 12 weeks was 3.4 points on the RMDQ scale, which was more than twice that of manipulation in the UK BEAM study among a similar group of patients and follow-up time.

Three other important research studies in the US (Kimberly Williams et al 2003, 2005, 2009) have found specialised Iyengar yoga classes to be effective. The 2009 trial followed 90 people for 48 weeks. The conclusion was that "Yoga improves functional disability, pain intensity, and depression in adults with chronic low back pain. There was also a clinically important trend for the yoga group to reduce their pain medication usage compared to the control group" (the control group = the non-yoga participants who received standard medical care). This trial found positive effects after 12 weeks for yoga classes; a further increase in beneficial effects after a further 12 weeks of yoga and a maintenance of these effects at 48 weeks.

The smaller yoga trials mentioned in this section all had limitations, e.g. only one teacher, but are nevertheless consistent with The University of York trial's findings with regards to improvements in back function.

Authors' Comments

From anecdotal evidence, yoga teachers believe that appropriate regular yoga practice helps to maintain the long-term health of the joints and musculature at the same time as improving outlook on life. It would be interesting to follow up people after many years of practising yoga for back health.

Yoga is more likely to have a long-term influence than, for example, manipulation, as yoga is self-empowering. It is something people learn to do for themselves. Students are asked to practise at home between classes and to continue well beyond their first course of lessons. Yoga teaches self-awareness. For instance, people who practise yoga are more likely to notice when they are undertaking a task, or perhaps sitting, in a way that is unhelpful to their spine or posture. Yoga also has the potential to strengthen mental health and to help avoid negative neurological cycles associated with pain.

References

Cox, H., Tilbrook, H., Aplin, J., Chuang, L-H., Hewitt, C., Jayakody, S., Semlyen, A., Soares, M.O., Torgerson, D., Trewhela, A., Watt, I., Gill Worthy, G.: A pragmatic multi-centred randomised controlled trial of yoga for chronic low back pain: trial protocol. *Complementary Therapies in Clinical Practice.* 2010. 16:76-80.

Lamb, S.E., Hansen, Z., Lall, R., Castelnuovo, E., Withers, E.J., Nichols, V., Potter, R., Underwood, M.R.: Group cognitive behavioural treatment for low-back pain in primary care: a randomised controlled trial and cost-effectiveness analysis. *The Lancet*, DOI:10.1016/S0140-6736(09)62164-4.

Little, P., Lewith, G., Webley, F., Evans, M., Beattie, A., Middleton, K., Barnett, J., Ballard, K., Oxford, F., Smith, P., Yardley, L., Hollingurst, S., Sharp, D.: Randomised controlled trial of Alexander technique lessons, exercise, and massage (ATEAM) for chronic and recurrent back pain. *British Medical Journal*, 2008: 337: a884.

Roland, M., Waddell, G., Moffett, K.J, Burton, K., Main, C.: 2002. *The Back Book*, 2e. The Stationary Office. First published 1996.

Sherman, K.J., Cherkin, D.C., Erro, J., Miglioretti, D.L., Deyo, R.A.: Comparing yoga, exercise, and a self-care book for chronic low back pain: a randomized, controlled trial. *Annals of Internal Medicine*, 2005. 143. 849-856.

Tilbrook, H.E., Cox, H., Hewitt, C.E., Chuang, L-H., Jayakody, S., Kang'ombe, A.R., Aplin, J.D., Semlyen, A., Trewhela, A., Watt, I., Torgerson, D.J.: Yoga for chronic low back pain: a randomized trial. *Annals of Internal Medicine*. (November 2011).

UK BEAM Trial Team United Kingdom back pain exercise and manipulation. UK BEAM randomized trial@effectiveness of physical treatments for back pain in primary care. *British Medical Journal*, November 2004.

Williams, K., Steinberg, L., Petronis, J.: Therapeutic Application of Iyengar Yoga for Healing Chronic Low Back Pain. *International Journal of Yoga Therapy No. 13* (2003) p.55

Williams, K., Petronis, J., Smith, D., Goodrich, D., Wu, J., Ravi, N., Doyle, Jr. E., Juckett, G., Kolar, M., Gross, R., Steinberg, L. Effect of Iyengar yoga therapy for chronic low back pain. *Pain* 115, 107-117, 2005.

Williams, K., Abildso, C., Steinberg, L., Doyle, E., Epstein, B., Smith, D., Hobbs, G., Gross, R., Kelly, G., Cooper, L. Evaluating of the effectiveness and efficacy of Iyengar yoga therapy on chronic low back pain. *Spine*, 2009, Vol.34, No.19 pp.2066-2076.

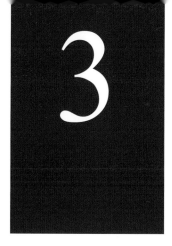

3

Resources for the *Yoga for Healthy Lower Backs* Course

The materials and resources referred to as part of the *Yoga for Healthy Lower Backs* course include:

- This *Yoga for Healthy Lower Backs* book
- The *Yoga for Healthy Lower Backs* Relaxations CD (see below) which is available as a CD by post from *www.yogaforbacks.co.uk*
- A yoga mat
- A yoga block or a book such as a telephone directory
- A yoga belt, ordinary belt or non-stretchy tie or scarf
- A firm blanket
- A pillow (or cushions). A yoga bolster or a fanned blanket may be used as a substitute for a pillow, when taught by qualified teachers in some pose variations
- A chair with a flat chair-seat and without chair-arms

If you do not already have these items, you may wish to consider purchasing them. As well as *www.yogaforbacks.co.uk* (funded by CD sales), *www. yogamatters.co.uk* is another source of yoga products, such as mats.

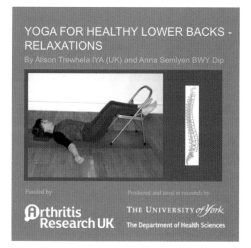

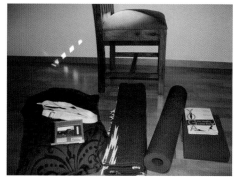

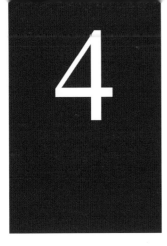

How to Find a Yoga Teacher

As yoga is a movement skill, it is strongly recommended that you get support to learn yoga. In short, that you pay for, and attend, an appropriate weekly yoga class or have private lessons.

Many yoga classes offered commercially by self-employed yoga teachers, or at gyms or by local authorities, will include posture work that is more demanding than is appropriate for someone with low back pain.

Ideally find a yoga teacher specifically trained in the *Yoga for Healthy Lower Backs* course. These are experienced teachers and are listed on *www.yogaforbacks.co.uk*. If there do not appear to be teachers near you, then perhaps ask your local yoga teachers to consider doing the *Yoga for Healthy Lower Backs* training course.

Please bear the following in mind when considering joining a yoga class.

Qualifications

- Check that the teacher is fully qualified to teach yoga and holds a current yoga teaching diploma and insurance.
- Ask about the teacher's qualification. We recommend teachers from the yoga organisations listed in Section 14, i.e. The British Wheel of Yoga and The Iyengar Yoga Association (UK). Both have high training standards.
- Ask about the teacher's training and experience in teaching therapeutic or remedial yoga for the low back. Are they also working as a yoga therapist?
- Have they completed the *Yoga for Healthy Lower Backs* full four-day training course? (see Section 15).
- If time allows, you could try contacting several yoga teachers and see who you like best as a person.

Style of Yoga Teaching

- Ask if the teacher runs *Yoga for Healthy Lower Backs* specialist classes. Once you have attended such a course, other suitable follow-on examples might be back care classes, foundation level classes or beginners' yoga classes.
- Ask about numbers of students in each class. In smaller size classes you will get more attention and a more individualised style of class.
- Ask about, or notice, the way that the teacher works. For instance do they appear observant? Do they walk around class checking the student's postures? How long is relaxation time?
- Ask if the teacher ever manually adjusts students. State the preference that you would like to be offered, verbal descriptions and demonstrations rather than hands-on adjustment, if that is what you prefer.

Prices

- Ask about class prices and any discounts for booking in advance. In some locations it may be possible to get some or all of the class fees paid for you by the NHS (yoga on prescription), your employer, or your private health insurance provider.
- Ask if you can try a trial class before committing to paying for a course of lessons. If you do like the class and teacher, then paying up front for a course of lessons will definitely help to motivate you to attend and is therefore recommended.
- Enquire whether the teacher does private lessons and the costs. If affordable, consider booking a one-to-one lesson before going to a class. The teacher will then be able to meet you personally. He or she may want to do an assessment; for instance by asking about the history of your back health. Some teachers will do some yoga diagnostics such as asking you to complete certain posture tests, for instance leg raising from lying on your back. A yoga therapist would be likely to want to visually look at your posture and back shape. A private lesson will give you time to listen and respond to any questions you may have relating to your needs, whether these concern your physical, mental or emotional health.
- At a class make sure that the teacher is aware of your health, that you have had, or are experiencing, back pain and tell them about any other relevant health conditions or if you become pregnant.

■ Ideally the teacher has yoga props, like blocks, to loan to students. Or you might decide to buy your own block to help with comfortable sitting and as a head support. A yoga mat will be useful as it will keep you warm and prevent you slipping.

The Venue and Timings

■ Ideally choose a class location that is close to where you live or work and at a time that suits your schedule. This makes getting there easier and you will be more likely to maintain regular attendance, but in reality it may be necessary to travel.

■ Ideally the venue is warm, quiet, has chairs and access to yoga use of the walls.

■ *Yoga for Healthy Lower Backs* courses that consist of 12 PROGRESSIVE classes will begin on a specific date, so be prepared to telephone to register and then wait until the next start date.

If You Are Experiencing Difficulty With Your Yoga Practice

■ Know that you are in control of your body. If the teacher demonstrates something in class that you do not feel is appropriate for your health or your back, then you may choose to relax or do something else in this manual instead. Participation is voluntary.

■ If, for any reason, you are not getting along with a yoga teacher or the venue, explain your problems or issues. He or she may be able to make useful changes to improve matters. For instance by making the room warmer, by helping you to be more comfortable using props such as blocks, or offering easier (or more challenging) modifications or variations to the poses.

■ If you decide to change classes, ask perhaps if your teacher can suggest a class with fewer students or a private session in order to give you more individual attention, or perhaps they can recommend another local teacher.

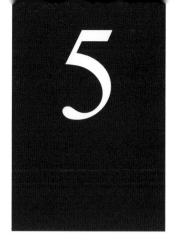

5 Committing to Yoga

Yoga aims to help you to be your own teacher; you are in control of your own movements and exercises. At a *Yoga for Healthy Lower Backs* class, yoga teachers will not usually make any physical adjustments to you. A teacher will explain verbally how to improve your posture or breath. Your own self-awareness will improve with yoga practice.

Preparing for Yoga

- Wear comfortable layers of clothing in which you can move and breathe freely.
- Have a firm blanket or rug and a belt (or tie or non-stretchy scarf).
- Practise when drug-free, including painkillers, and sober.
- Go to the toilet before doing yoga.
- It is best not to practise with a full stomach.
- If you have a teacher, tell him or her about any concerns in changes to your health or if you become pregnant.
- Align yourself to be square with the walls.
- Practise slowly, with awareness and with the breath.
- Do not be concerned if you feel some muscular aches after class, much as athletes in training do when they are improving their physical fitness.
- Exercise so as to avoid exacerbating leg pain during and after the yoga.
- Ask a teacher for help if you have difficulty following the yoga or are not feeling comfortable.
- Some poses are best done in bare feet. An alternative for a cold room is to wear socks with non-slip soles.

Home Practice

- This is something you do for yourself, so enjoy this empowering feeling of self-help.
- This is your time, so ensure that you will not be disturbed – find a quiet, warm room and switch off the phone.
- Do the exercise sequences you have been taught regularly at home, referring to the *Suggested Home Practice Timetable* to be sure you are practising the correct sequence.
- Practise the yoga slowly and steadily.
- Breathe steadily throughout your yoga.
- Remember it is not what you do, but the way that you do it. Be attentive at all times.
- If you don't get on with a particular posture, leave it out for now or imagine yourself doing it in your mind only, but do ask a teacher about possible adjustments and refinements, because it could be the very posture you need most.
- Always listen to your body and ease off/stop the posture if you meet pain and use this new awareness in your everyday life. Be aware of your body more of the time.
- Lie and practise relaxation. Listen to the companion educational resource *Yoga for Healthy Lower Backs* Relaxations CD regularly. Relaxation is as important as physical yoga practice.
- Enjoy your home practice sessions. You could try practising at a different time of the day.
- It is good to allow yoga awareness to spill into your daily life. Observe and correct your breath, posture and mental state throughout your day.
- Keep a positive attitude and remind yourself often that you DO want to improve. The body wants to be healthy, but you need to encourage it to be so.
- Make a note of your home practise and progress in a notebook.

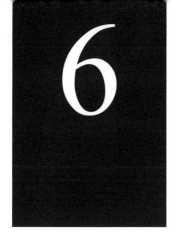

6 Yoga for Your Daily Life

- **Defy gravity**: Stand tall; lift up; find height; lift chest and top of head; un-crumple trunk; feel confident, worthy and strong.

- **Find more symmetry**: Stand evenly on your two feet; use your arms and legs more similarly and evenly; equal length to both sides of your trunk; head straight; find more symmetry in daily activities, e.g. don't always sit the same side on to breakfast bar.

- **Good posture more often**: Feet parallel; strong legs; correct pelvic alignment; correct natural curves to spine; open chest; relaxed shoulders.

- **Breathe well**: Observe and encourage a steady even breath more of the time; quality inhalations to bring your energy levels up; quality exhalations to relax and calm; deeper breath to enliven brain to its full potential.

- **Power of the exhalation**: Purposeful steady exhalations to relieve pain; to perform awkward movements; to lift; to lessen muscle tension; to calm the mind.

- **Relaxed face**: Tension in the facial muscles is often a reflection of tension in the body and/or the mind, so remind the face to relax, especially around the organs of perception/senses (eyes, ears, mouth, nose, throat, tongue, skin). Relax the forehead, temples, jaw and back of the skull.

- **Live more in the present**: Yogis spend more time in the present – noticing the weight on the feet, the breath, emotional reactions and preventing tension build-up – and so they experience more of their life in reality. Being in the present more of the time – less depression about the past or anxiety about the future – allows life and time to stop rushing by and allows one to look at oneself. This can bring more life satisfaction, more creativity and more productivity and allows one to view life from a positive new perspective.

▨ **Notice and reinforce the good times**: Mental attitude is important: aim to observe yourself and thereby lessen annoyance, depression, anxiety, self-defeatism, doubt, fear, etc. Appreciation of positive sensations and comfort in your body are important, as research suggests that small amounts of positive in our lives can far outweigh large amounts of negative. Turn your 'OK day' into 'the best day ever' by savouring the taste of a delicious raspberry or the sight of a beautiful sunset or how comfortable your body feels after your yoga practice.

Advice On Daily Activities

▨ It is good to vary body position if possible, so don't sit for hours without a break.

▨ Try some of the following as shown by your yoga teacher during your course and find what works for you.

Sitting

Sofa: use cushions behind lower back and upper back; length on front of body; avoid slouching.

Hard chair: clench buttock muscles and brace abdominal muscles on exhalation; place a hand on abdomen to lift it in and up; sit evenly on both buttocks and backs of thighs; have feet level; if crossing legs, make sure both crosses are done for the same amount of time.

Computer: adjust the chair; sit squarely and upright; if looking at documents, turn to both sides not just one side; take regular stretch breaks (hourly), e.g. shoulder and arm stretches or leg stretches.

Driving: rolled/fanned towel as a lumbar support; say "Ahhhh" a few times to bring pelvic tone and relax muscle tension; on an exhalation clench buttock muscles and brace abdominal muscles; sit evenly on both buttocks and backs of thighs; imaginary use of left leg as per right foot's pedal work to make pelvis feel even.

Arising From Sitting

Feet flat and firm; lift chest; brace abdominal muscles; strong legs; lead with top of head; arise on exhalation and inhale once standing.

Bending Down

Maintain straight back; bend more from knees and hips; execute bend on exhalation; come up straight and not from the side.

Standing

Sit down or squat down for relief; stand as Mountain Pose; stand evenly right and left; lift up arches of feet and kneecaps; abdomen in and up; symmetry to legs and pelvis; turn toes in; 'dinosaur tail' (tailbone down behind); 'jeans pockets' (back of pelvis down and around to sides;) hands on abdomen to take in and up; poise; defy gravity; tie belt around pelvis (for sacroiliac stability and abdominal support for lumbar).
Cleaning teeth/washing up: Try one foot up on a raise, e.g. low stool or under-sink cupboard (alternate feet); one hand on abdomen to hold it in towards the spine; brace abdomen.

Walking

Same as standing; lift arches of feet; carry in both arms or alternate arms.

Shopping/tourism: strong legs with lifted kneecaps; weight in heels; pelvis above front ankles not over toes.
For exercise: outer legs firm; even stride right and left; as Mountain Pose; stretch calf/quadriceps/hamstrings if unevenly stiff.
Uphill: lift chest; strong legs especially outer thighs and quadriceps.
Downhill: tuck tailbone down and in; abdomen back in place.

Cough/Sneeze

Brace abdomen; hand on abdomen; brace buttocks.

Housework

Strong arms, legs and abdominal muscles; exhalations for effort; firm outer thighs and buttocks when turning during vacuuming; when reaching up bring in abdomen and tailbone; TBR (Table-Top Back Relaxer) for relief.

Lying

On front: use pillow lengthwise under chest, abdomen and pelvis and progress to widthways pillow under pelvis and/or abdomen.
On back: use yoga relaxation positions as shown; firm surface is best for yoga, but pad with even blanket under if necessary.
In bed: exhale to turn over; do yoga relaxation in your head; count your exhalations by counting backwards slowly from 20 to 0 becoming more relaxed with each number; breathe and exhale as if through the skin at tense or painful areas.
On side: pillows under top leg or between legs; fanned small towel under bottom side of waist; lie along pillow from waist to head; plump up pillow under side neck leaving less under ear/side of head; pillow directly behind you; diagonal pillow under head and behind neck and shoulders.

Gardening

All fours for weeding; use both hands; exhale to lift; perform SIS (Sacroiliac Stabiliser) after overdoing gardening work.

Sport

Exhale on effort, e.g. to hit ball; strong legs, strong arms and strong abdominals; use yoga to aid flexibility, strength and mental focus.

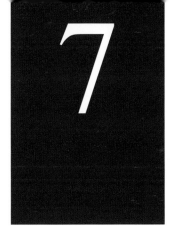

What to Do If You Get a Sign of a Painful Back Episode

Pain Prevention – Pain Relief

These poses can act as natural pain-relievers; you should choose just one. They are definitely best performed having learnt them under the guidance of a knowledgeable teacher, and they constitute positions where the body and mind can feel completely passive and at ease – you should therefore not experience any tension, worry or a sensation of stretch.

You may like to record in pencil which poses helped you to feel better and when. Bear in mind that your favourite effective pose this month may not be the same pose next month or next year. To find out more about the benefits of these poses, follow the maroon **Page Numbers** referring to full descriptions in Section 10, but bear in mind that there may be slight differences to be sure that these are completely restful for body, back and mind.

1. Don't panic!

2.   Do at least 15 minutes of **Yoga Relaxations** on the floor listening to the Relaxation CD.

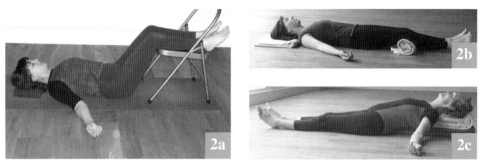

a.   On back; calves on chair-seat; book/folded blanket under head and neck; *most useful pain-relieving position for majority of back conditions*. **Page 128.**

b.   On back; knees bent over pillow/rolled blanket; support under head and neck. *useful for disc problems*. **Page 128.**

c.   On back; sit on floor and lie spine from waist up along lengthwise pillow; book/folded blanket on top of pillow under head and neck; legs straight (as shown in photo) OR calves on chair-seat; *useful for sciatica, disc problems or sacroiliac discomfort.* **Page 132.**

3.   Adopt just ONE of these **Relief Poses** slowly, gently and comfortably and concentrate on breathing steadily, focusing on the **relaxing exhalations**. Timings given are maximum, so don't overdo it – in this instance, these are not stretches. **Exhale to enter and exit pose. Easy, comfortable, pain-free.**

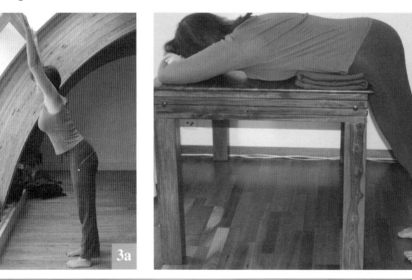

a. **STRETCH ARMS UP HIGH TO WALL OR LEDGE** (30 seconds); *after slouchy sitting (in car or sofa).* **Page 68.**

b. **TABLE-TOP BACK RELAXER (TBR):** lie pelvis and chest onto table with pillow/blanket under abdomen; resting forehead onto folded arms; legs may be bent (facets/muscles) or walked back towards straight (discs) (4 minutes); *great for all back/brain/neck aches.* **Page 60.**

c. **CHAIR-SEATED FORWARD BEND** from hips to rest forehead on folded arms supported by table; keep length on front of body; change arm cross half way through (3 minutes); *after sitting upright (at desk), long periods of standing or twisting awkwardly.* **Page 58.**

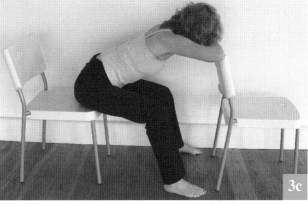

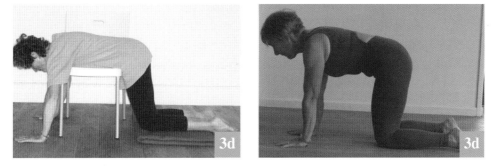

d. **ALL FOURS Kneeling**: can gently rock forward and back (2 minutes). This can be done over chair; *after straining back, e.g. lifting.* **Page 101.**

e. **SACROILIAC STABILISER (SIS):** lying on tummy; forehead on fingers with elbows bent out to sides; tuck toes under and firm legs and buttocks (20 seconds x 3). Relax well after each repetition, especially in buttock area, with toes in/heels out; *after overdoing the gardening/ forward-bending and for sacroiliac joint symmetry.* **Page 111.**

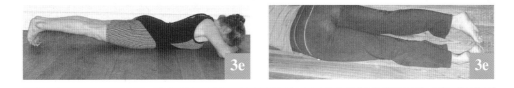

f. **LYING TWISTS**: on back; knees bent; feet hip-width apart; arms at 45° to sides – take knees to side, i. 6 inches only; *iliopsoas rebalance*, ii. halfway down, iii. as far as is comfortable (5-10 seconds each side); *after back feels stiff/tight*. **Page 113.**

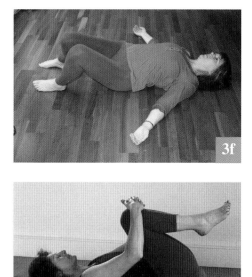

g. **DOUBLE LEG LOCK**: on back; hold knees to chest; can gently, i. bring knees in and out or, ii. gently rock from side to side (4 minutes); *after travelling and if muscles are sore.* **Page 124.**

4. Be especially aware of your posture, movements, sitting position. Aim to relieve tension and **don't challenge your back for a few days.**

5. Don't despair, but learn from the build-up, recovery and rehabilitation.

6. Keep positive and know that you can help yourself.

7. After 1 or 2 days of doing the above, return gently to your usual yoga session, provided it is pain-free.

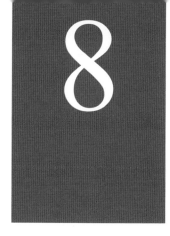

Yoga Sequences

Introduction

These are some of the most important pages of the manual as they give you a shortened version of the yoga sequences you will be following at home. It is important to follow a sequence for optimum effect, but leave out or do an 'imaginary' pose, if some poses do not suit you.

Please refer to Section 10 to remind yourself how to perform the pose and for finer details or observations. You can easily refer to the relevant page in Section 10 by following the coloured page numbers shown at the end of each short text description. *N.B. When following CORE practise sequences, make sure you only do the simpler versions of the pose – directly underneath the green pose name heading above the photograph in Section 10, it must be listed as Refs: CORE (followed by the relevant pose number).*

Within a 12-class *Yoga for Healthy Lower Backs* course you will be given the following sequences during the class week shown in brackets:

- ■ 'What to Do If You Get a Painful Back Episode' pain-relieving pose sheet plus '*Yoga for Healthy Lower Backs* Relaxations CD' (Week 1)
- ■ **CORE Practice A** (Week 2)
- ■ CORE Practice B (Week 3)
- ■ COMPLETE CORE Practice (Week 6)
- ■ **PROGRESSIVE Practice A** (Week 7)
- ■ **PROGRESSIVE Practice B** (Week 8)

(N.B. The numbering is correct even if there seem to be some numbers missing.)

The **CORE Practices** will give you the tools to maintain the health of your lower back now and in the long-term. You are encouraged to practise especially the **CORE A** sequence at least twice a week and we hope you will be inspired to practice it forever (even if only eventually once a week).

The **PROGRESSIVE Practices** include many of the yoga poses from the **CORE Practices**, and add more poses that will build on the understanding you have gained.

As everyone has a different body and a different starting-point, and each of us learns and progresses at our own speed, some may find that practising the **CORE Practices** mostly and the **PROGRESSIVE Practices** only occasionally is better. Others may find that it feels best later on when the back feels stronger to practise the two **PROGRESSIVE Practices** alternately. The 'Suggested Timetable of Daily Yoga Practice for Healthy Lower Backs' (9) is an example only and you should aim to find what works best for you.

Be led by your own body and mind. Leave out anything that does not feel right and ask your teacher for advice.

Find a regular time to practise daily – the optimum time (for your back) would probably be the middle of the day – but find a time that suits you best.

Please enjoy your yoga.

CORE A

CORE Practice A

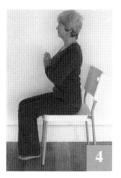

4. **CHAIR-SEATED + PALMS TOGETHER**
   Closed Eyes
   i.   **PELVIC-FLOOR-UPS & TUMMY-INS** *x 3.*
   ii. **"AHH"S** *x 3.*
   Page 79.

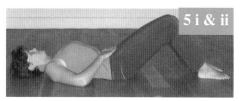

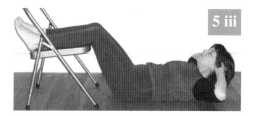

5. **LYING PELVIC TILTS**
   i.   **ACTIVE** (use abdominal
        and buttock muscles) *x 3.*
   ii. **PASSIVE** (use leg muscles)
        x 3.
   iii. **ABDOMINAL CURL-
        UPS** + calves on chair-seat
        x 3.
   Pages 82–84.

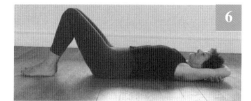

6. **FRONTAL BODY STRETCH**
   Knees bent; fold arms overhead
   x 2 folds *1 minute.*
   Page 92.

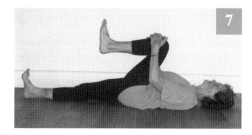

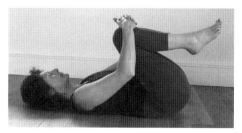

7. **SINGLE LEG LOCK**
   One knee into chest.
   Pages 97–98.

DOUBLE LEG LOCK
Knees to chest after.
Page 124.

CORE A

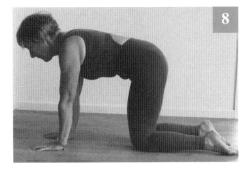

8. **ALL FOURS**
   Kneel on all 4s (still or rock gently forwards and back) *30–60 seconds.*
   Page 101.

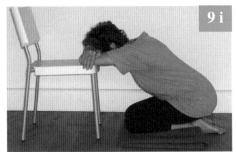

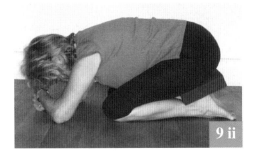

9. **POSE OF CHILD**
   Sit to heels, knees slightly apart
   i.   Rest forehead onto folded arms on chair-seat *60 seconds.*
   ii. Forehead on hands on floor (You may be advised to leave this out) *60 seconds.*
   Page 103.

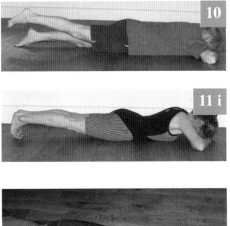

10. **PRONE SINGLE LEG LIFTS**
    (Tailbone in) *x 1–3*, hold each repetition for 1 breath.
    Page 108.

11. **SACROILIAC STABILISER SIS**
    i.   Prone, toes tucked under, forehead on hands, firm legs *x 2 10 seconds.*
    ii. Relax well after; toes in/ heels out.
    Page 111.

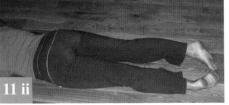

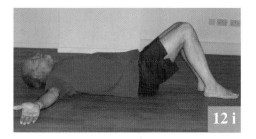

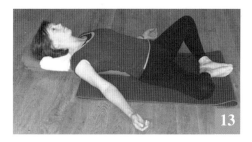

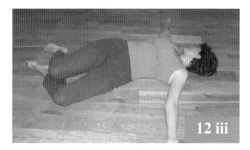

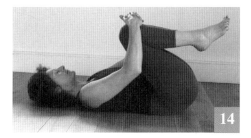

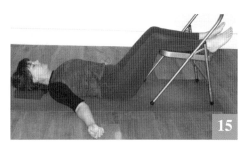

12. LYING TWISTS
Knees bent, feet on floor and hip width apart, left then right
i.   **TILT** both knees only 4 inches to one side *30 seconds.*
ii. **STEADY MOVEMENT IN AND OUT** – knees down on exhale, up on inhale; smooth movement and breathe *x 10.*
iii. **FEET HIP DISTANCE, HOLD, WITH HEAD TURN** Knees down to side and hold, with head turned opposite way *15–30 seconds.*
Pages 113–116.

13. RECLINED COBBLER POSE
Lying along pillow from waist; book/folded blanket on top of pillow under head and neck; soles of feet together; knees out (onto supports for comfort) *1 minute.*
Page 121.

14. DOUBLE LEG LOCK
On back; knees to chest
i.   **JELLY WOBBLE** (knees gently in and out)
ii. **SPINAL ROCK** (rock from side to side)
iii. **STILL**
All versions 30–60 seconds.
Pages 124–125.

15. SAVASANA – RELAXATION
(Relaxations CD)
5–10 minutes.
Pages 128–131.

CORE Practice B

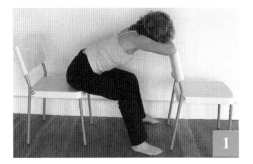

1. CHAIR-SEATED FORWARD BEND
Bend forward from hips; forehead on folded arms on table/ledge *1–3 minutes*.
Page 58.

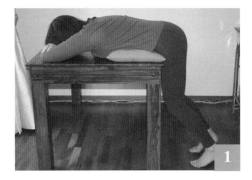

OR **TABLE-TOP BACK RELAXER TBR**
Lie trunk forward onto table-top; forehead on folded arms (blanket under abdomen) *1–3 minutes*.
Page 60.

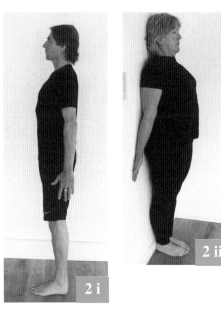

2. MOUNTAIN POSE
i.   Strong, firm and steady away from wall *30 seconds*.
ii. Back to wall 20 *seconds*.
Page 65.

3. **SHOULDER STRETCHES**
   i. **STRETCH ARMS UP HIGH TO WALL OR LEDGE**
      10 seconds.
   ii. **ARMS UP FROM SIDES TO OVERHEAD** Inhalation: take arms up, palms facing up; exhalation: take arms down, palms facing down *x 5*.
   iii. **ARMS UP FROM FRONT TO OVERHEAD** Palms forwards *10 seconds*.
   iv. **HUG ARMS AND BENT KNEES** *x 2* crosses of arms *10 seconds*.
   Pages 68–72.

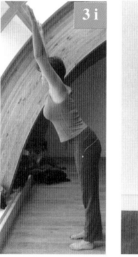 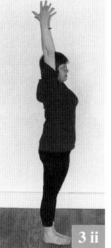 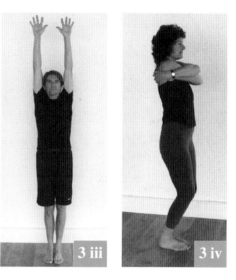

3 i   3 ii   3 iii   3 iv

15. **SAVASANA – RELAXATION**
Relaxations CD *5–15 minutes*.
Pages 128–134.

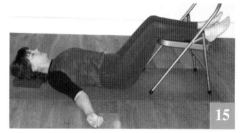

15

Complete *CORE* Practice

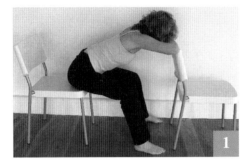

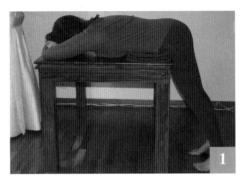

1. **CHAIR-SEATED FORWARD BEND**
   Bend forward from hips; forehead on folded arms on table *1–3 minutes*.
   Page 58.

OR **TABLE-TOP BACK RELAXER**
   Lie trunk forward onto table-top; forehead on folded arms (blanket under abdomen) *1–3 minutes*.
   Page 60.

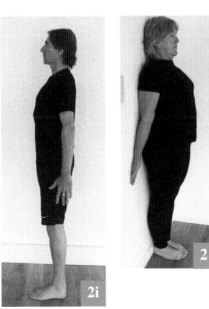

2. **MOUNTAIN POSE**
   i.   Strong, firm and steady away from wall *30 seconds*.
   ii. Back to Wall 20 *seconds*.
   Page 65.

3. **SHOULDER STRETCHES**
    i.   **STRETCH ARMS UP HIGH TO WALL OR LEDGE**
         10 seconds.
    ii. **ARMS UP FROM SIDES TO OVERHEAD** Inhalation: take arms
         up, palms facing up; exhalation: take arms down, palms facing down
         x 5.
    iii. **ARMS UP FROM FRONT TO OVERHEAD** Palms forwards
         10 seconds.
    iv. **Hug Arms and Bent Knees** *x 2* crosses of arms *10 seconds.*
    Pages 68–72.

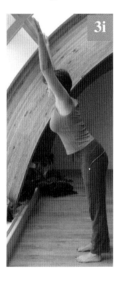
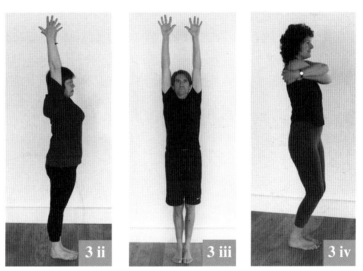

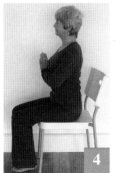

4. **CHAIR-SEATED + PALMS TOGETHER**
    + Closed Eyes
    i.   **PELVIC-FLOOR-UPS AND TUMMY-INS**
         x 3.
    ii. **"AHH"S** *x 3.*
    Page 79.

CORE

5. **LYING PELVIC TILTS**
    i.   **ACTIVE** (use abdominal and buttock muscles) *x 3*.
    ii. **PASSIVE** (use leg muscles)
         x 3.
    iii. **ABDOMINAL CURL-UPS** + calves on chair-seat *x 3*.
    Pages 82–84.

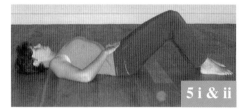

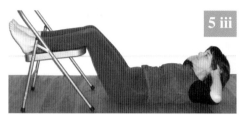

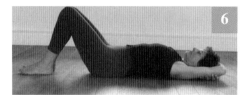

6. **FRONTAL BODY STRETCH**
    Knees bent; fold arms overhead
    x 2 folds *1 minute*.
    Page 92.

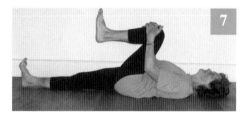

7. **SINGLE LEG LOCK**
    One knee into chest *30 seconds*.
    Pages 97–98.
    DOUBLE LEG LOCK
    after
    Page 124.

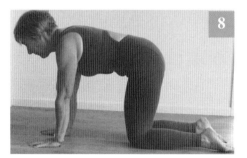

8. **ALL FOURS**
    Kneel on all 4s (still or rock
    gently forward and backward)
    30–60 seconds.
    Page 101.

9. **POSE OF CHILD**
    Sit to heels, knees slightly apart:
    i.   Rest forehead onto **FOLDED ARMS ON CHAIR-SEAT** *60 seconds*.
    ii. **FOREHEAD ON HANDS ON FLOOR** You may be advised to leave this out *60 seconds*.
    Page 103.

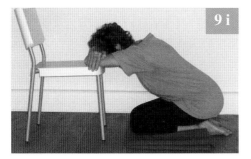
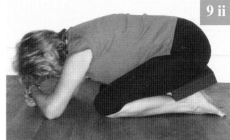

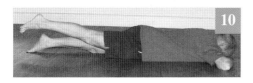

10. PRONE SINGLE LEG LIFTS
(tailbone in) *x 1–3*, hold each repetition for 1 breath.
Page 108.

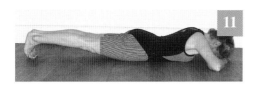

11. SACROILIAC STABILISER
SIS Prone, toes tucked under, forehead on hands, firm legs *x 2 10 seconds*. Relax well after; toes in/heels out.
Page 111.

12. LYING TWISTS
Knees bent, feet on floor and hip width apart, left then right
i.   **TILT** both knees only 4 inches to one side *30 seconds*.

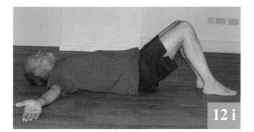

ii. **STEADY MOVEMENT IN AND OUT** – knees down on exhale, up on inhale; smooth movement and breathe *x 10*.

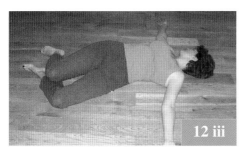

iii. **FEET HIP DISTANCE, HOLD, WITH HEAD TURN** Knees down to side and hold, with head turned opposite way *15–30 seconds*.
Pages 113–116.

CORE

CORE

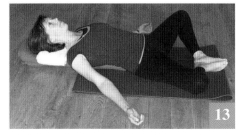

13. **RECLINED COBBLER POSE**
Lying along pillow from waist; book/folded blanket on top of pillow under head and neck; soles of feet together; knees out (onto supports for comfort)
1 minute.
Page 121.

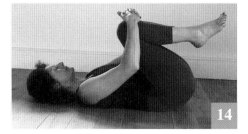

14. **DOUBLE LEG LOCK**
On back; knees to chest
  i. **JELLY WOBBLE** (knees gently in and out)
  ii. **SPINAL ROCK** (rock from side to side)
  iii. **STILL**
All versions 30–60 seconds.
Pages 124–125.

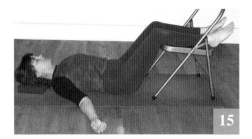

15. **SAVASANA – RELAXATION**
(Relaxations CD)
5–10 minutes.
Pages 128–131.

PROGRESSIVE Practice A

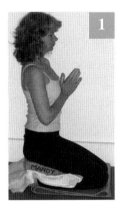

1. **BEGINNING/SETTLING POSES**
    i.   **KNEELING, PALMS TOGETHER**
          "AUM"S – *x 3*, sit to heels (or in chair).
    Page 62.

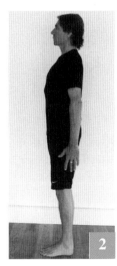

2. **MOUNTAIN POSE**
    Check from feet to head *30–60 seconds*.
    Page 65.

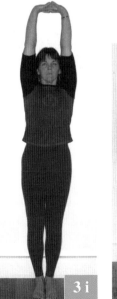

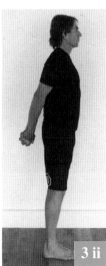

3. **SHOULDER STRETCHES**
    i.   **OVERHEAD
          INTERLOCK** Interlock
          fingers; stretch palms
          overhead *15 seconds*.
    ii.   **INTERLOCK BEHIND**
          Interlock fingers; arms
          straight behind back (hold
          belt?) *15 seconds*.
    Pages 73–75.

PROGRESSIVE A

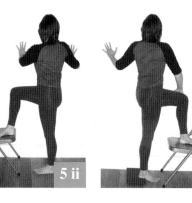

5. **CHAIR TWISTS**
   ii. **STANDING CHAIR TWIST**
   Side on to wall; turn toward foot up on chair-seat; place hands on wall (**on second variation**: standing foot **HEEL UP** on block; **HAND TO KNEE**) *10–15 seconds*.
   Page 90.

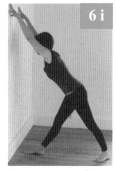

6. **STANDING POSES**
   i. **FORWARD STRETCH OVER ONE LEG**
   Fingertips to wall; both legs straight; one leg forward and other leg backward, 3 feet behind; straight back *15–20 seconds*.
   Page 94.

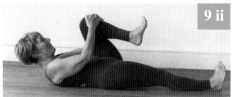

7. **ABDOMINAL POSES**
   ii. **LYING SINGLE LEG RAISES** Other leg bent, 30°, 60°, 80° up with alternate legs; lift on exhalations *x 1–3*.
   Page 86.

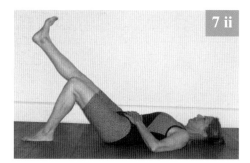

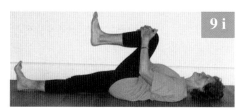

9. **SUPINE HIP AND LEG STRETCHES**
   i. **SINGLE LEG LOCK.** Lying; one knee held to chest *30–60 seconds*.
   ii. **SINGLE LEG LOCK WITH HEAD LIFT.** Lift head on exhalation *10 seconds*. **Page 97.**

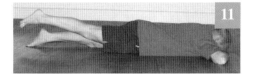

11. PRONE POSES
   i. **PRONE SINGLE LEG LIFTS**
      Tailbone in; pelvis down *x 3*. **Page 108.**

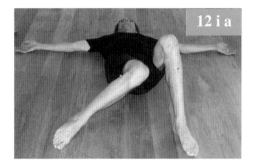

12. LYING TWISTS
   Feet on floor; knees bent; legs down on exhalation, left then right 30 *seconds* each.
   i. **FEET WIDE,**
      a. **ONE KNEE IN,**
      b. **BOTH KNEES DOWN.**
   ii. **LEGS CROSSED** – down toward bottom knee side.
Page 117.

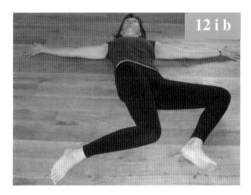

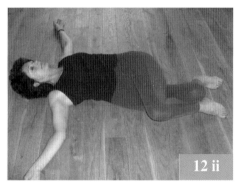

14. DOUBLE LEG LOCK
   Hold knees to chest.
   i. **CIRCLE KNEES**
      Hands on knees, twice each way *x 3*.
      STILL hold after *30 seconds*. **Page 126.**

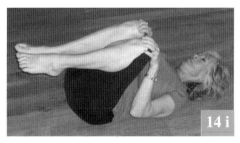

15. SAVASANA – RELAXATION
(use CD once a week) *5–20 minutes* (sometimes with Pranayama – breathing awareness).
Page 128.

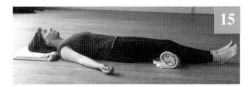

PROGRESSIVE Practice B

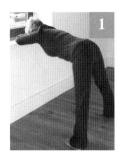

1. **BEGINNING/SETTLING POSES**
   ii. **FOLDED ARMS TO LEDGE/CHAIR-BACK**; feet 1 to 3 foot apart; toes turned in, *1 minute*.
   Page 64.

3. **SHOULDER STRETCHES**
   iii. **HEAD OF COW**
      Catch belt behind back; one elbow up and other elbow down *10–15 seconds*.
   iv. **EAGLE POSE**
      Entwine arms in front; bend legs *10–15 seconds*.
   Page 76.

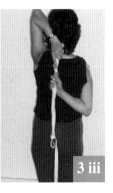

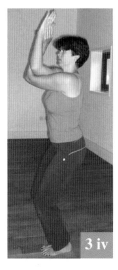

4. **HANDS TO WALL BACK STRETCH**
   Feet parallel and hip distance *15–30 seconds*.
   Page 81.

5. **CHAIR TWISTS**
   i. **SEATED CHAIR TWIST**
      Sit side on; hold chair-back; turn from waist up *x 2* *10–15 seconds*.
   Page 88.

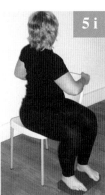

PROGRESSIVE B

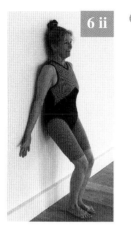

6. **STANDING POSES**
   ii. **IMAGINARY CHAIR POSE**
        Back to wall; feet 9 inches from wall; knees
        bent *15–20 seconds*.
   Page 96.

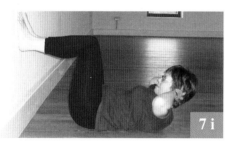

7. **ABDOMINAL POSES**
   i. **ABDOMINAL CURL-
       UPS
       BOAT POSE**
       Lying with feet boxed to
       wall; fingers holding head
       by ears; exhale lift up/
       inhale down; slow *x 3*.
   Page 85.

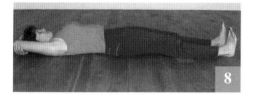

8. **FRONTAL BODY STRETCH
   – LEGS STRAIGHT**
   Lying on back; knees bent;
   fold arms above head *x 2*
   folds. Stretch legs straight, **if
   comfortable** *30–60 seconds*.
   Page 92.

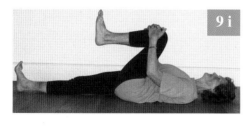
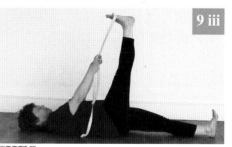

9. **SUPINE HIP AND LEG STRETCHES**
   iii. **SINGLE LEG LOCK then HAMSTRING STRETCH**
        Knee to chest; belt on foot; straighten leg up *20–30 seconds*.
   Pages 97 and 100.

PROGRESSIVE B

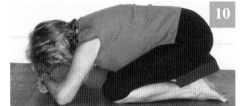

10. POSE OF CHILD
Sit to heels; bend forwards from hips; head resting; use supports (e.g. chair) as necessary. *1–2 minutes*.
Page 105.

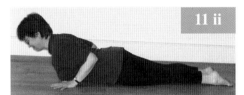

11. PRONE POSES
ii. **COBRA POSE**
Prone; strong legs; tailbone in; low lift *10–15 seconds*.

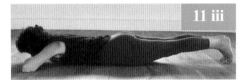

iii. **SACROILIAC STABILISER SIS + HEAD LIFT**
Prone with toes tucked under; firm legs; lift head 4 inches *x 2 10–20 seconds*. Relax well after; toes in/ heels out *1 minute*.
Page 109.

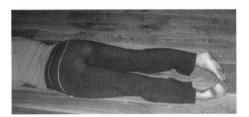

12. LYING TWISTS
Feet on floor; legs down on exhalation left then right
iii. **FEET TOGETHER**
x 2 30 seconds.
Page 119.

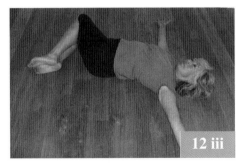

13. RECLINED COBBLER POSE
Lying (along pillow?); soles together; knees out; arms to sides; support legs as necessary; with comfort *1–3 minutes*.
Page 121.

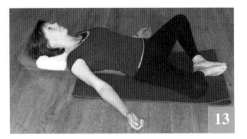

PROGRESSIVE B

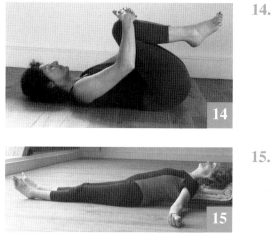

14. **DOUBLE LEG LOCK**
    Hold knees to chest
    ii. **SPINAL ROCK**
        Rock gently from side to
        side 1 minute
        Still hold *30 seconds*.
    Page 124.

15. **SAVASANA – RELAXATION**
    (use Relaxations CD once a
    week) *5–20 minutes* (possibly
    with **PRANAYAMA** –
    breathing awareness).
    Page 128.

During Week 1 you are firstly aiming to learn how to gain some comfort and calm in your body and your mind, as well as learning how to fit home practise into your daily life. For Week 1, the following practise timetable requires you to JUST ONE pain relief or pain prevention pose from Section 7 and follow that with a yoga relaxation (using track 1 of the CD).

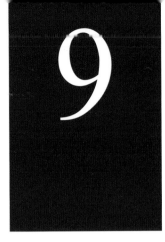

Suggested Timetable of Daily Yoga Practice for Healthy Lower Backs

Every Person is Different

This is a guide to be used in conjunction with a 12-class *Yoga for Healthy Lower Backs* course including a 2 week mid-course break.

If you find the **CORE Practice** is helping you best, use this more often, instead of including the **PROGRESSIVE Practices**.

If you are not on a course or if you miss classes or do not have time to practise, then you will need to postpone moving on throughout the suggested weeks of the timetable.

While you are aiming to make real changes to the health of your back, you will benefit from the discipline of practising as per this timetable, but once your back feels stronger and you feel more flexible and confident, then you can aim to maintain back health by practising twice a week.

During Week 1 you are firstly aiming to learn how to gain some comfort and calm in your body and your mind, as well as learning how to fit home practice into your daily life. For Week 1, the following practice timetable requires you to try JUST ONE pain relief or pain prevention pose from Section 7 'What to Do If You Get a Sign of a Painful Back Episode' and follow that with a yoga relaxation (using Track 1 of the 'Yoga for Healthy Lower Backs–Relaxations' CD.)' You will find the short CD tracks useful to use in isolation or after your yoga practice and especially if you have had an uncomfortable or stessful day.

Class 1	Day 1	Day 2	Day 3	Day 4	Day 5	Day 6	Day 7
Week 1	"What To Do If..." 3a + Relaxations CD Track 1	"What To Do If..." 3b + Relaxations CD Track 1	"What To Do If..." 3c + Relaxations CD Track 1	"What To Do If..." 3d + Relaxations CD Track 1	"What To Do If..." 3e + Relaxations CD Track 1	"What To Do If..." 3f + Relaxations CD Track 1	"What To Do If..." 3g + Relaxations CD Track 1 Class 2
Week 2	CORE A	CORE A	CORE A	CORE A	CORE A	Relaxations CD Track 1	Class 3
Week 3	CORE B Relaxations CD Track 2	CORE A	CORE B Relaxations CD Track 1	CORE A	CORE B Relaxations CD Track 2	Relaxations CD Track 1	Class 4
Week 4	CORE B Relaxations CD Track 3	CORE A	CORE B Relaxations CD Track 4	CORE A	CORE B Relaxations CD Any Track	Relaxations CD Any Track	Class 5
Week 5	CORE A	CORE B	CORE A	CORE B	CORE A or B	Relaxations CD Any Track	Class 6
Class Break Week 6	CORE A	CORE B	CORE A	CORE B	CORE A	Relaxations CD Any Track	CORE
Class Break Week 7	CORE A	CORE B	CORE A	CORE B	CORE A	Relaxations CD Any Track	CORE
Week 8	CORE A	CORE B	CORE A	CORE A or B	CORE B	Relaxations CD Any Track	Class 7
Week 9	PROGRESSIVE A	CORE B	PROGRESSIVE A	CORE A	PROGRESSIVE A	Relaxations CD Any Track	Class 8
Week 10	PROGRESSIVE B	CORE B	PROGRESSIVE A	CORE	PROGRESSIVE B	Relaxations CD Any Track	Class 9
Week 11	PROGRESSIVE B	CORE	PROGRESSIVE A	CORE	PROGRESSIVE B	Relaxations CD Any Track	Class 10
Week 12	PROGRESSIVE A	CORE	PROGRESSIVE B	CORE	PROGRESSIVE A or B	Relaxations CD Any Track	Class 11
Week 13	PROGRESSIVE A	CORE	PROGRESSIVE B	CORE	PROGRESSIVE A or B	Relaxations CD Any Track	Class 12
Week 14-52	CORE	PROGRESSIVE A	CORE	PROGRESSIVE B	CORE	Relaxations CD Any Track	Other Yoga Class?

Keep Up Your Yoga. You Owe It To Yourself.

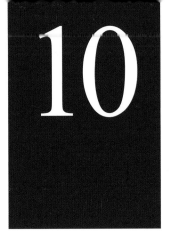

10 Long Descriptions of Yoga Poses

Introduction

This section will be invaluable to yoga teachers and existing yoga students.

The descriptions of the yoga poses in this section are designed for use once one has been shown and taught them in class. Throughout a 12-class *Yoga for Healthy Lower Backs* course, yoga students are introduced to practice sequences at appropriate times. By all means read bits of this chapter whenever you like, but do not attempt to perform all the poses unless you are referring to the practice sequences in Section 8 – this will tell you which order to follow, as well as the length of time or how many repetitions to do.

Some people like knowing lots of information, whilst others may feel overloaded by being given too much. It is not necessary to use all the information on these pages, but they may be very useful from time to time and especially when practising at home after the 12-week course has finished.

If you are attending a *Yoga for Healthy Lower Backs* Course, use the 'Suggested Timetable of Daily Yoga Practice for Healthy Lower Backs' (Section 9) to remind yourself of which particular sequence you should be practising during a particular week. If you are not attending such a taught course, then you will be likely to take much longer to grasp a full understanding of the sequences effectively – this will mean practising the CORE sequences for longer (or possibly until you find a teacher).

Yoga is an art, a science and a philosophy and it is best learnt from a teacher, but these pages will help to remind you of the poses in your practice sequences and should help to stimulate your enthusiasm for yoga practice.

Photographs

At first we learn yoga best visually, so refer to the photograph, which should remind you of how the teacher looked when demonstrating and how you felt when in the pose. Without a class, you will need to study the photograph and the text carefully.

Pose Names and Reference Numbers

When practising a particular home practice sequence (as recommended by your teacher), you can find the name of the yoga pose and the reference number here, e.g. Pose of Child – Adho Mukha Virasana is No. 9 on the CORE Practice sequence and No. 10 on the PROGRESSIVE Practice sequence.

We have chosen English pose names that we feel will allow you to readily differentiate which pose we mean, but yoga was originally documented by the ancient language of Sanskrit (with its own script) and we have included the Sanskrit name in this section too.

How to Perform the Pose

This is a basic description of how to enter and exit the yoga pose. Refer also to your practice sequence page for appropriate timings.

Observations

Once we know basically how to perform the pose, we can pay attention to sensations and experiences whilst performing the yoga. The points given in this section will vary in type and include some instructions that your teacher may have given you in class plus a few new ones.

They may be instructions or observations:
- to make the pose more comfortable.
- to make the pose more effective.
- to bring mental focus.
- to observe the effects of the pose and reactions whilst in the pose.

■ to learn more precision to bring your body and mind more into tune.
■ to notice more layers of subtlety.
■ to keep you interested in performing the same poses over future years.

You may like to read one or two of these observation points and then aim to incorporate them into your practice of the pose. They may prove very useful if you become bored with, unsure of, or unconvinced by a particular pose.

Some will be more useful to you than others. Of course, your teacher is the best source of information and can usually help you more than written words, so please ask them for clarification whenever necessary.

Variations

These variations will include many that a teacher will teach you on a 12-class *Yoga for Healthy Lower Backs* Course. Some use props (pillows, chairs, walls, etc.) to make the pose more accessible and/or more effective. Some will help to emphasize a certain aspect of the pose. Some will make the pose easier and some harder and they will add interest to your practice.

Benefits

Many extra physical and mental benefits have been experienced from each pose, some of which are listed in this section. Added incentives to practise!

Related Yoga Poses

Once you have completed your 12-week course, you may one day want to join a 'Beginners', 'General' or 'Foundation' Yoga class and it may interest you to refer to this small section to find which poses have similarities to your own vault of self-knowledge. The majority of the poses you will learn in this yoga programme also have useful links to each other.

Index

To find a particular pose, please refer to the index of poses at the end of this book.

The Cross of Learning

One of the wonderful aspects of yoga is that the subject is vast. Learning can take place at various levels and layers and go in various directions. Typically in the West, we feel we must learn 'vertically' with learning becoming more difficult as we go in an upward direction. Similarly, we can learn more challenging yoga poses, but the more yoga we do, often the more we benefit from returning to the very basic, simple poses and penetrating downward or inward gaining more precision, depth and subtlety. In yoga we also learn 'horizontally', by adding ever more details about the same poses. All these different directions of learning should be regarded as progression in yoga.

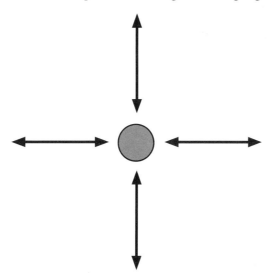

CHAIR-SEATED FORWARD BEND – *Pavanamuktasana*
Refs.: CORE No.1   What To Do If... No. 3c

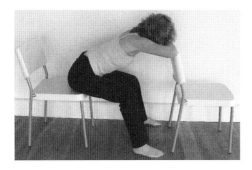

How to Perform the Pose
With a high table/ledge in front of you, sit at the front of a hard chair-seat, placing your feet flat on the floor with your feet wider than your hips and heels underneath your knees. With your hands placed firmly on your top front thighs, inhale and lift up your spine. On an exhalation, hinge forwards from your hips, keeping length and space on the front of your trunk, i.e. no crinkles on the front of your clothing and space from pubic bone to navel to front ribs. Place your elbows on the table/ledge and rest your forehead in your hands. (**You may stay here if this suits you better and you are experiencing any sciatica or leg symptoms.**) If this feels comfortable, fold your arms with your elbows no wider than shoulder distance apart and place them a little further forwards on the table. On an exhalation gently rest your forehead onto your arms. Stay and relax here for up to 3 minutes. To exit the pose: on an exhalation gently lift your head and use the strength of your arms to bring you upright in the chair, keeping your back muscles uninvolved and relaxed. Inhale once you are upright. Change the arm cross halfway through the time held, either whilst in the pose or exit and re-enter.

Observations
- This is a forward bend and not a downward bend, so bend from the hips and not from the waist.
- **The aim of this position is to rest and relieve the back and brain; there should not be a great stretch on the back muscles. If too much stretch, bring the arms higher (a book on the table or a higher ledge) and/or sit closer forwards.**
- It is important to pay attention to any leg symptoms. If sciatic pain or other leg symptoms are experienced in this pose or after this pose, leave it out for now and tell the teacher.
- Encourage the forehead skin to smooth down from hairline to eyebrows; rather than the other way around, as this is more relaxing.
- Experience the breath and just 'be' in the present moment.

▥ Encourage the shoulders, shoulder blades and trapezius muscles to move down the back in order not to crowd out the neck; let the back of the neck be long and soft.

Variations

■ For sciatica or other leg symptoms, leave this out and try Table-Top Back Relaxer (see next pose) with legs far back behind instead.

■ When experienced, try bending forwards from hips (with front of body long and no rounding of the back), starting with hands on the front thighs by the knees and then placing elbows onto knees with palms together.

Benefits

✓ Teaches how to sit comfortably.

✓ Lengthens and relaxes paraspinal muscles, thereby pacifying and relieving lower back muscle spasm and backache.

✓ Opens up and gently stretches facet joints.

✓ Relaxes the mind and the muscles of the head and face.

✓ Relieves headaches.

Related Yoga Poses

Adho Mukha Virasana, Uttanasana, Paschimottanasana.

TABLE-TOP BACK RELAXER (TBR)
– *Salamba Ardha Uttanasana*
Refs.: CORE No. 1   What To Do If… No. 3b

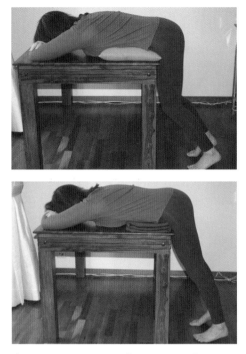

How to Perform the Pose
With feet hip distance apart, stand in front of a firm, high table (or breakfast bar/chest of drawers). On an exhalation and without exaggerating the curve in your lower back, place the front of your pelvis and abdomen onto the table-top and gently lower yourself onto your elbows. On another exhalation, stretching your armpits, rest your folded arms on the table and rest your forehead on them. Your elbows should be no wider than shoulder distance apart. Depending on the height of the table, you may need to bend your knees (lower table) or stand up on tiptoes (higher table) to get into this pose. Once in the pose, you can have your legs straight, but more usually bent; you may walk your legs further backwards so that you are on tiptoe with straight legs (especially for those with disc-related sciatica). Rest and relax in this position for up to 3 minutes or more. To exit the pose: on an exhalation, gently lift up your body and head using the strength of your arms and keeping the back muscles uninvolved and relaxed and avoiding exaggerating the curve in your lower back. Inhale once you are standing upright. Change the fold of the arms halfway through.

Observations
- This should be a gloriously relieving and relaxing pose for all cases of low back pain, so enjoy it.
- Encourage the forehead skin to smooth down from hairline to eyebrows, rather than the other way around for extra relaxation.
- Experience the breath and just 'be' in the present moment.

■ Encourage the shoulders, shoulder blades and trapezius muscles to move down the back in order not to crowd out the neck; let the back of the neck be long and soft.

■ The back muscles may enjoy a gentle stretch as well as a rest, which can be achieved by slowly bending the knees little by little until the optimum sensation is felt.

■ Notice how the abdomen is back in place, the pelvis is level and symmetrical, the back muscles are long and relaxed and the brain is quiet.

Variations

■ Try placing a pillow or evenly folded blanket under the pelvis and abdomen for cushioning and/or to lessen the lordotic curve of the lower back (especially good for 'sway-back' and/or facet joint problems).

■ Try over a tall piece of furniture where the arms and head relax over the end (for more advanced practice).

Benefits

✓ Pain-relieving pose for the lower back (almost all conditions); horizontal offloading effect on all the structures of the back without the need to get down on the floor or to put pressure on any sensitive parts of the back.

✓ Relaxes the musculature of the whole back of the body, whilst at the same time giving stable support at the front.

✓ Opens up and gently stretches the facet joints.

✓ Offloads the sacroiliac joints (thereby giving relief from strain and/or pain).

✓ Gently stretches the back muscles, as well as the shoulder and neck muscles.

✓ Relieves tension headaches and pains in the neck and reduces nervous tension.

✓ Pacifies a nervous stomach or bowel; can reduce palpitations.

✓ Beginning forward bend with space for discs at front of spine.

Related Yoga Poses

Uttanasana, Virabhadrasana III.

KNEELING, PALMS TOGETHER 'AUM'S
– *Vajrasana and Namaskarasana*
Ref.: PROGRESSIVE No. 1i

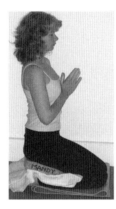

How to Perform the Pose

Sit to your heels in a kneeling position, making absolutely sure your knees are comfortable (see below). Bring the palms together in front of your chest in a prayer position, with the base of the palms level with your lower breastbone and your elbows out to the sides. Close your eyes. Prepare with a complete exhalation, take an inhalation deep into your abdomen and then on the out-breath make the sound of "Aum". Take a recovery breath or two and repeat x 3.

Observations

- If uncomfortable in the knees, place a ½ to 1 inch thick folded blanket into the back of the knees and one or more books or firm cushions on top of the heels and under the buttocks (in photo above). **If still unable to be comfortable in the knees, sit in a chair.**
- If the front ankles are uncomfortable, place a rolled blanket or a pillow under the front of the ankles.
- Allow the heels to go out comfortably.
- Root the tailbone down to prevent overarching the lumbar as you lift the spine up.
- Lift the breastbone forwards and up towards the hands; the energy of the heart ascending.
- Balance the head erect above the spine.
- Stretch the fingers up and slightly forwards; have the thumb away from the fingers and pointing up and touching the centre of the breastbone.
- Relax the eyelids and imagine the energy of the brain descending downwards on the exhalations.
- Keep the upper arms away from the side ribs and the inner elbows descending.
- Relax the shoulders down encouraging the sides of the neck to relax.
- Allow the skin of the palms to melt into one another, without pressing.
- Allow the diaphragm to spread and move down and the ribcage to expand on the inhalation.

- The sound should not be as an opera singer, but should emanate from the belly as a rich sound that rises upwards.
- During the sound, the mouth should be wide and gradually become more and more closed until the 'Mm' at the end.
- Keep the jaw relaxed.
- Do not strain.
- For varicose veins, use chair-seated version instead.

Variations
- Try an "Ahh" (pelvis), then an "Ouhh" (chest), then an "Mmm" (head), before putting the sounds together and observe the different vibrations and the emphasis on different parts of the body.
- Make a loud sound, or a softer quieter sound, or even just whisper the sound.
- Sit in a chair.

Benefits
- ✓ Comfort for the lower back (as on a kneeling chair).
- ✓ Stretches the front ankles and the feet, encourages higher arches to the feet and lessens heel spurs.
- ✓ Brings flexibility to the knees, but if this does not come comfortably to start with, know that lying on the back with knees to chest, Double Leg Lock will bring flexibility without weight-bearing for the healthy flexion of arthritic knees.
- ✓ Relaxes the lower back muscles and encourages a natural lumbar curve.
- ✓ Calms and rests the brain: closing the eyes allows the brain approximately 40% rest.
- ✓ Relaxes the shoulders and neck, whilst lifting the spine.
- ✓ Teaches lengthening of the breath: a deep inhalation followed by a longer relaxing, calming exhalation.
- ✓ Centres the mind for mental focus; the mind will follow the sound.
- ✓ Good beginning practice at the start of a yoga session as it brings physical and mental balance and equilibrium.

Related Yoga Poses
Virasana, Sukkhasana, Siddhasana, Padmasana.

FOLDED ARMS TO LEDGE – *Ardha Uttanasana*
Ref.: PROGRESSIVE No. 1ii

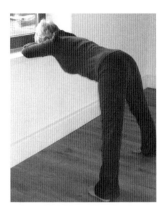

How to Perform the Pose
Stand in front of a ledge approximately 4 feet high (window sill, table, chair-back), with your feet parallel and 1–3 feet apart. On an exhalation place your hands, then your elbows onto the ledge and fold your arms. With the arms resting on the support, rest your forehead on your arms. Turn your toes in; have your legs straight and your back rested and straight. Stay and relax for up to 1 minute. Change the fold of the arms halfway through.

Observations
■ The ledge support should be of a comfortable height: if it is too high, bring the legs closer together; if it is too low bring the legs wider apart.
■ Adjust the foot position backwards so that the back feels comfortably stretched and rested and the front of the body is long.
■ The bend comes from the hips, not the waist.
■ Keep the elbows at shoulder distance by holding the upper arms.
■ Take the shoulder blades and trapezius muscles down the back and maintain length at the back of the neck.
■ Encourage the skin on the forehead to move downwards from the hairline to the eyebrows.
■ Enjoy the comfort this pose gives to the back.
■ Relax the brain.

Variations
■ Go higher and have the feet together.
■ Go lower onto the chair-seat and have the feet very wide.
■ Try folding arms overhead first (when stronger).

Benefits
✓ Offloads the structures of the back, bringing comfort to the sacroiliacs, facet joints, muscles, tendons and ligaments.
✓ Calms and rests the brain.
✓ Relieves anxiety; relaxes the diaphragm.
✓ Brings a feeling of equanimity and equilibrium.

✓   May help to control blood pressure.
✓   Relieves and prevents hot heads (hot flushes, anger, stress, headache).

Related Yoga Poses
Uttanasana, Prasarita Padottanasana, Tadasana, and Baddha Hastasana.

MOUNTAIN POSE – *Tadasana*
Refs.: CORE No. 2   PROGRESSIVE No. 2

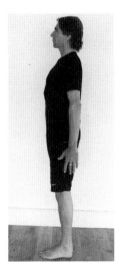

How to Perform the Pose
Stand with your feet together, joining the inner edges of your feet from big toe joint to inner heels. Lift the arches of your feet. Lift your kneecaps by engaging your quadriceps (front thigh muscles). Draw your outer thighs inwards, bringing the heads of your femur bones into the hip joints. Draw all the muscles of your legs upwards. Tuck your tailbone in and up. Draw your lower abdomen and navel in and up. Lift your breastbone forwards and up, allowing your shoulders to relax back and down. Lift the crown of your head up while pressing the soles of the feet down into the ground. Gently stretch your arms and hands. Breathe steadily. Stand still for up to 1 minute.

Observations
▪ Have even weight on all 4 corners to both feet, neither allowing the knees to become knocked or bowed; especially keep the weight over the front of the heels.
▪ Be square with the room as with all your yoga poses.
▪ Avoid the tendency to push the pelvis and front thighs forwards and the compensatory leaning back of the trunk, which will exacerbate lower back pain.
▪ Aim to spread the toes and do not turn your feet out.
▪ Relax the mouth, jaw and tongue, which if tense can exacerbate low back tension.
▪ Note how important this learning experience of how to stand is in relation to everyday life and also to many of the other yoga poses.
▪ Be especially aware to correct any tendency to rotate the pelvis to one side (use a wall close in front to measure).

- Make sure both legs are evenly straight and have the weight evenly on both feet.
- Find as much symmetry as possible everywhere, e.g. not pushing one hip out to the side; equal length on both sides of the waist.
- Make sure the head is not tilted to one side and aim to have the shoulders level.
- Find the correct pelvic position where it is neither tilted forwards nor back.
- Defy gravity.
- Feel strong.
- Be aware of how both the abdominal and leg strengthening help to lift the body up off the lower back for height, space, lightness, poise and relief.
- As the body lifts, the spirits lift.
- As the heart lifts, the mood elevates and confidence increases (light-hearted).
- Learn to stand on "your own two feet" (literally and metaphorically).

Variations and Benefits
See below after Mountain Pose with Back to Wall.

MOUNTAIN POSE WITH BACK TO WALL – *Tadasana*
Ref. CORE 2ii

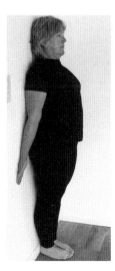

How to Perform the Pose
Stand with your back against a wall (heels to the wall if possible). Take your tailbone down the wall and bring your abdomen in and up. Use your hands to teach the abdomen to move in and up. Lift your breastbone up and spread your collarbones to the sides. Encourage the back of your head to go towards the wall without lifting the chin and without strain. Place the backs of your hands on the wall, turning your arms out. Stay for up to 20 seconds. Note where your body is now with this alignment teacher.

Variations

- Stand with the feet under the hips.
- Lie on the back and try a lying version of this pose. Maybe have the feet flat against a wall as though your feet were in a standing position.
- Tie a tight belt around the sacrum for sacroiliac stability (ask your teacher).
- Do this correct standing posture often throughout the day.

Benefits

- ✓ Teaches correct standing technique and good posture.
- ✓ Gives relief in many cases of backache that are caused by postural imbalance.
- ✓ Slows and lessens degeneration of the whole skeletal system if performed with balance, symmetry and alignment (less arthritis).
- ✓ Good posture is efficiency.
- ✓ Gives optimum space for the organs for their health, e.g. a slumped saggy abdomen is less likely to have healthy intestines and bowel and a collapsed chest will not help to maintain healthy lungs and heart.
- ✓ This pose teaches the foundation to many yoga poses.
- ✓ Useful for everyday life. Notice how you stand anywhere and everywhere.
- ✓ Strengthens the body.
- ✓ Focuses the mind.
- ✓ Pain relief now and for the future as correct posture is found, improved and maintained.

Related Yoga Poses

Samasthiti; all yoga poses.

SHOULDER STRETCH – STRETCH ARMS UP HIGH (TO WALL) OR LEDGE – *Urdhva Hastasana*
Refs.: CORE No. 3i   What To Do If … No. 3a

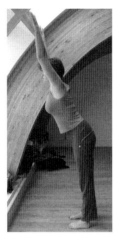

How to Perform the Pose
Ledge Variation: Stand 1–2 feet away from and facing a high ledge, e.g. the top of a doorframe or the top of a stable piece of furniture that is taller than you. Instructions as below in Wall Variation but place your fingers onto the ledge and use it to give the tractioning effect of gentle hanging, but with your feet firmly on the floor and legs straight and upright. Hold for 10 seconds and exit the pose on an exhalation.

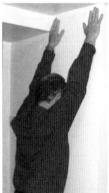

Wall Variation: Stand approximately 1 foot away from and facing a wall with your feet hip distance apart and feet parallel (or slightly turned in). On an exhalation reach your arms up high to place the palms of your hands flat on the wall; hands shoulder distance apart with stretched armpits and straight arms. Your legs should be perpendicular to the floor with the weight in your heels and you should feel an upwards elongation to your trunk, especially the front of your body.

Observations
- Keep a comfortable neck: by taking the outer armpits forwards towards the wall; keep the neck in line with the spine; take the trapezius and shoulder blades down the back; lengthen the neck and head out of the shoulders.
- Feel the stretch on the sides of the trunk: armpits, side ribs, side waist.
- Take the outer side hips out into the middle of the room.
- Mountain Pose legs.
- Maintain the natural curve in the lumbar region, but realise that this pose can help to lessen the exaggerated curves that can occur in the spine, e.g.

lessen the roundedness of the upper back and lessen the inward curve of the lower back by paying attention to it (there should not be a large back-bending hollow and in the lumbar region the spine should not have disappeared into a deep ravine).

Variations

- Turn toes in a lot to stabilise the spine.
- Turn hands out (when using the wall) and/or take them wider for stiff shoulders.

Benefits

- ✓ Encourages mobility in the upper back and shoulders and teaches more mobility in those areas and less in the lumbar region.
- ✓ Beneficial space for the discs at the front of the spine.
- ✓ Traction effect for stiff spinal segments (but more stable than 'hanging' from bar/beam).

Related Yoga Poses

Virabhadrasana I, Adho Mukha Svanasana, Adho Mukha Vrksasana.

SHOULDER STRETCH – ARMS UP FROM SIDES TO OVERHEAD – *Urdhva Hastasana*
Ref.: CORE No. 3ii

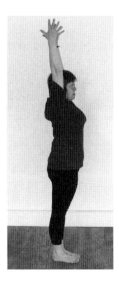

How to Perform the Pose

Stand in Mountain Pose and on an inhalation, with your palms facing upwards, take your arms straight up from the sides to overhead until the palms touch. On an exhalation, with your palms facing downwards, take your arms down by the sides. Repeat up to 5 times.

Observations

■ Try keeping the arms relaxed and soft (as if going through feathers) and then try keeping the arms and hands firm and active (as if going through treacle).

■ Avoid the tendency to take the weight towards the toes and to take the pelvis forwards: keep the weight in the heels and the pelvis back over the heels.

■ Take the arms to a place where the shoulders are not strained: if necessary take the arms slightly forwards and/or not quite to the top.

■ Make the breath steady and smooth and notice how the upward movement of the arms encourages the movement of the inhalation from deep down within the abdomen and on up into the top chest.

■ Breathe through the nose (as always) and avoid sucking the nostrils inwards.

■ Observe how the body gains height as the arms lift upwards.

■ Keep the legs strong, especially pressing the feet downwards on the inhalation.

Variations

■ Keep the palms facing down, lift to shoulder height; then turn palms up by rotating at the shoulder joints and take arms overhead; with palms facing up bring arms down to shoulder height, turn palms down and continue to bring arms down to sides (teaches more specific shoulder action).

Benefits

✓ Deepens and lengthens the breath in a relaxed way. This is energising for the brain.

✓ Brings height to the trunk.

✓ Preparatory strengthening of the musculature of the trunk.

✓ Mobility in the shoulders.

✓ Unifies the breath, the mind's focus and the bodily movements.

Related Yoga Poses

Vrksasana, Virabhadrasana I.

SHOULDER STRETCH – ARMS UP FROM FRONT TO OVERHEAD – *Urdhva Hastasana*
Refs: CORE No. 3iii

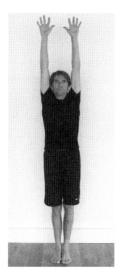

How to Perform the Pose
Stand in Mountain Pose. Take your arms out in front of your body with your palms facing down. Keep your shoulders pressed down with the shoulder blades anchored down the back. On an exhalation, keeping the weight back in the heels, take your arms overhead with your palms facing forwards. Hold for up to 10 seconds, lifting up more on the inhalation and then bring your arms down from the front.

Observations
- Maintain the strength of the legs.
- Continue to breathe steadily.
- Don't overstay.
- Look straight ahead and keep the chin up a little (especially for neck comfort).

Variations
- Take one arm up only (can lean slightly over to side to get even more lateral stretch – reach arm diagonally up to ceiling).

Benefits
✓ As Arms up from Sides to Overhead, but better understanding of inner shoulder action rather than outer and increased strengthening of the back trunk.

Related Yoga Poses
Adho Mukha Vrksasana, Adho Mukha Svanasana.

SHOULDER STRETCH – HUG ARMS AND BEND KNEES – *Garudasana* Variation
Ref.: CORE No. 3iv

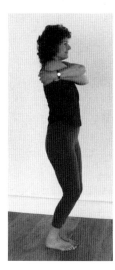

How to Perform the Pose
Stand in Mountain Pose. Put your arms straight out in front of you with the palms together. Inhale and open your arms out to the sides. On an exhalation bring your arms hugging around your body, elbows crossed and right arm over the top of the left. On another exhalation bend your knees. Hold for up to 10 seconds. Exit the pose on an exhalation by straightening your legs and undoing the arms. Repeat with your left arm on the top.

Observations
- Relax the shoulders down.
- Observe the space in the back of the chest, but keep comfort at the front chest.
- Breathe into the back of the shoulders to relieve any tension there.
- Observe the space between the shoulder blades.
- Enjoy the hug and be kind with the hands.
- Keep the heels down and no need to bend the knees very far, as the Achilles tendon and calf muscles will restrict, (do not bounce).
- Have the head above the tailbone, i.e. have an upright trunk.
- Encourage the tailbone to feel heavy and to sink down behind and the muscles of the lower back to move downwards from the waist.
- Encourage the inner thighs/groins to move down and back, the outer thighs to move forwards and the sacral area at the back of the pelvis to broaden from the centre to around the sides of the pelvis.
- Feel comforted and valued.
- Allow the knees to touch lightly.

Variations

- Later on: progression to eagle pose arms (PROGRESSIVE Practice 3iii).
- Perform several repetitions of opening the arms out to the sides on the inhalations and to bring the arms into a hug on the exhalations to deepen the breath and wake up the brain.

Benefits

- ✓ Releases tension in the upper back and back of shoulders (rhomboids and trapezius muscles).
- ✓ Helps prevent tension headaches.
- ✓ Teaches good pelvic alignment, especially if one has a tendency to sway the back.
- ✓ Broadens the sacral area, thereby giving relief to compressed sacroiliac joints and discouraging piriformis muscle tightness.
- ✓ Stretches the calves.

Related Yoga Pose

Utkatasana.

SHOULDER STRETCH – OVERHEAD INTERLOCK
– Urdhva Hasta Baddhangullyasana
Refs.: PROGRESSIVE No. 3i

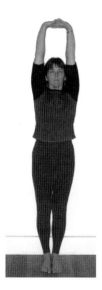

How to Perform the Pose

Stand in Mountain Pose with your feet together. Interlock your fingers, turn your thumbs down to stretch your arms in front of you with the palms facing forwards. On an exhalation, take the arms up overhead. Hold for up to 15 seconds. Release the interlock and take the arms down via the sides on an exhalation. Repeat with the other interlock, i.e. the other little finger at the back and the other thumb in the front.

Observations

- ▨ Keep the weight back towards the heels, but keep the toes spread and down.
- ▨ Maintain a natural curve in the lumbar region; do not take the pelvis forwards and arch the lower back; do not take the shoulders back either.
- ▨ In order to maintain the correct posture within the trunk, for stiffer shoulders it is better to keep the arms slightly forwards of upright, until flexibility comes with practice.
- ▨ Keep the legs strong, lift the arches of the feet and lift the kneecaps.
- ▨ Straighten the elbows and lift the wrists high.
- ▨ Keep length to the neck by anchoring the inner shoulder blades down and stretching the outer shoulder blades and armpits upwards.
- ▨ On the inhalations stretch up a little more.
- ▨ Keep the chin up and look straight ahead.
- ▨ As the arms stretch up, so the trunk responds with height and lift.
- ▨ The legs support from below and the arms lift from above for anti-gravitational poise and height.

Variations

- ■ If the wrists or fingers are stiff, hold the fingers of one hand with the other instead of interlocking.
- ■ To learn the comfort of the neck and shoulder blade action, take the hands onto the head with elbows bent to the sides first and then straighten the arms whilst anchoring the inner shoulder blades down and 'intending' the elbows to stay wide as straightening them.
- ■ Hold a book or a foam block overhead.
- ■ Sit in a chair for this shoulder stretch and learn to root the tailbone down.
- ■ Lie on the back on the floor for this shoulder stretch and learn to keep the pelvis in alignment.

Benefits

- ✓ Stretches the shoulders and upper trunk.
- ✓ Strengthens the back muscles.
- ✓ Brings flexibility to the upper trunk to reduce overuse of the lower trunk.
- ✓ Defies gravity – brings lift, height and space to the trunk and spine.

Related Yoga Pose
Parvatasana.

SHOULDER STRETCH – INTERLOCK BEHIND
– Paschima Baddhangullyasana
Refs.: PROGRESSIVE No. 3ii

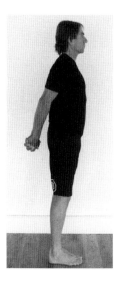

How to Perform the Pose
Stand in Mountain Pose with your feet together. Interlock your fingers behind your back and, with elbows bent, place your hands at the back of your pelvis with your thumbs on your sacrum. Broaden your collarbone area by taking your shoulders back and on an exhalation, keeping your palms facing towards your body, gently straighten your arms behind you as far as is comfortable. Hold for up to 15 seconds. Release your hands. Repeat with the other interlock of hands (your other thumb in front).

Observations
- Keep the weight in the heels.
- Take the armpit of the chest forwards and the armpit of the arm back.
- Feel the shoulders relaxing downwards away from the ears.
- Notice how the shoulder blades move closer together and how the muscles of the back move compactly and strongly towards the spine.
- Observe the openness of the chest.

Variations
- Hold a belt behind the back if your elbows cannot easily straighten.
- Sit at the front of a chair and hold the lower chair-back with straight arms.
- Have a looped belt on your wrists.
- Lie prone and perform the arm position.

Benefits
- ✓ Stretches the pectoral and biceps muscles.
- ✓ Strengthens the back of the shoulders to prevent rounded shoulders.
- ✓ Strengthens and brings tone to the backs of the arms.
- ✓ Brings a feeling of exhilaration.
- ✓ Improves lung capacity for healthy complete breathing.

Related Yoga Poses
Paschima Namaskarasana.

SHOULDER STRETCH – HEAD OF COW
– *Gomukhasana*
Ref.: PROGRESSIVE No. 3iii

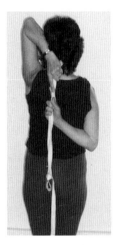

How to Perform the Pose
Stand in Mountain Pose with your feet together. On an exhalation take your straight right arm behind you, lift the chest, roll the arm in and, while bending your elbow, take the right hand up the back comfortably between the shoulder blades. Stretch your left arm up holding a belt and on an exhalation, bend your elbow to give the belt to the right hand. If you can comfortably do so, walk your left hand down the belt to catch the fingers of your right hand. Hold for up to 15 seconds. Release on an exhalation. Rest for a breath or two, before repeating on the other side.

Observations
- **If this pose feels too intense, leave it out and know that the other shoulder stretches are taking one towards this ultimate shoulder stretch.**
- Allow the bottom arm to feel warm in its straight back preparatory position, before taking it up behind the back.
- Keep the shoulder back when taking the bottom arm in.
- Use the other hand to aid the direction of the bottom hand up the back.
- Allow the head and neck to remain undisturbed by the top arm.
- Keep the elbow high as the top arm reaches down.
- Roll the top elbow in and up.

- Breathe through the shoulders to the elbows in order to release tension.
- Observe how the hands are encouraging the thoracic spine to move in and the chest to open.
- After releasing the arms, relax the shoulders well.
- Never be competitive in yoga, so do not catch the fingers if it causes strain.

Variations
- Learn the top arm action separately by holding the upper arm and turning it in.

Benefits
- ✓ Releases tension in the shoulders, upper back and neck.
- ✓ Prevents rounded shoulders.
- ✓ Prevents tension headaches.
- ✓ Encourages deeper breathing.
- ✓ Tones the arms.

Related Yoga Pose
Paschima Namaskarasana, Urdhva Hastasana.

SHOULDER STRETCH – EAGLE POSE
– *Garudasana*
Ref.: PROGRESSIVE No. 3iv

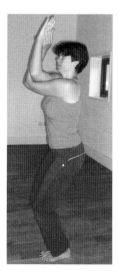

How to Perform the Pose
Stand in Mountain Pose with your feet together. Cross your arms in a hug across your chest and then keeping your elbows crossed, on an exhalation entwine the arms so that you can catch the fingers of your opposite hand in front of your face. Keeping your heels down, on an exhalation bend your knees. Hold for up to 15 seconds. Exit the pose and repeat with the other cross of arms.

Observations

- Keep comfortable space in the chest and comfort in the shoulders.
- If it is uncomfortable in the shoulders, either try using a belt or stay with the hugging position.
- Relax the shoulders down.
- Aim for the hands to be up above the elbows.
- Slowly bend the knees and keep the heels down.
- Have the knees touching lightly.
- Encourage muscles on the back of the pelvis to move downwards and the skin on the back of the pelvis to spread to the sides.
- Take the tailbone down.
- Encourage the outer thighs to move forwards as the inner thighs and groins move in and down.
- Maintain an upright spine with the head above the tailbone.
- Bring the abdominals lightly in and up.

Variations

- Stay with the hugged arms.
- Try this arm position lying on the back.

Benefits

- ✓ Reserves energy.
- ✓ Releases tension at the back of the shoulders and between the shoulder blades and the spine.
- ✓ Stretches the calf muscles.
- ✓ Has been used to improve peripheral vision.

Related Yoga Poses

Utkatasana, Malasana.

CHAIR-SEATED AND PALMS TOGETHER
– *Namaskarasana*
Ref.: CORE No. 4

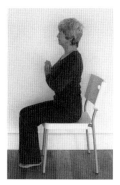

How to Perform the Pose

Sit towards the front of a firm chair-seat, with your feet parallel, under your knees and hip distance apart. Both feet must be firmly on the floor or supported on a block or book if needed. Bring your palms together in front of your chest in prayer position and close your eyes.

Observations

- Sit evenly on both sit-bones.
- Feet parallel and symmetrical.
- Relax the shoulders thereby allowing the sides of the neck to release.
- Have the spine and trunk lifted with the natural curves, but root the tailbone into the chair-seat to avoid overarching the lower back.
- Aim to have both sides of the trunk stretched up and of equal length.
- Lift the breastbone forwards and up using the support of the shoulder blades.
- Allow the skin of the palms to be open and the fingers straight, but avoid pressing the hands.
- Keep the elbows open and the collar-bones broad to allow the breath to move in the side rib area.
- Keep the eyelids and facial muscles soft.
- Relax the brain downwards on exhalations.

– PELVIC FLOOR-UPS AND TUMMY-INS
Ref. CORE No. 4i

How to Perform the Pose

Whilst seated in a chair as above, on an exhalation, pull up your pelvic floor muscles (toilet muscles from pubic bone to anal sphincter) and then at the same time encourage your abdominal muscles to pull in and up. Hold for a second or two. Repeat x 3.

Observations
- Feel as if this action starts with a gentle plugging in of the tailbone and then rises upwards to behind the navel.
- Take a breath or two between repetitions.
- Keep the face relaxed.
- Observe the strength and support on the lower front of the body.

Variations
- Aim to engage just the pelvic floor, as this will already involve the lower abdominals (good initial preparatory exercise).

– SAY "AHHHH" X 3
Ref.: CORE No. 4ii

How to Perform the Pose
Whilst seated in a chair as above, exhale fully and take a deep breath starting the breath from below your navel. On an exhalation, open your mouth wide and make the sound of "Ahh" until the exhalation is complete. Take a few normal breaths and then repeat twice more.

Observations
- Observe the vibration of sound within the lower trunk area.
- Be content with the sound made today.
- The mind will become focused on the sound and so this is being 'in the present moment'.
- Be relaxed in the mouth, jaw and throat.

Variations
- Sometimes try making a loud guttural sound and another day a small sound.
- If not appropriate to make a vocal sound, try opening the mouth to make a long steady sigh instead.
- Throughout the course of several weeks, try the sound of "Ouhh" (chest) and "Mmm" (head).

Benefits
- ✓ Symmetry and comfort in a seated position.
- ✓ Pelvic floor and abdominal strength, offering support to the lumbar spine.
- ✓ Postural education – tailbone action and pelvic alignment.
- ✓ Increased breathing capacity.
- ✓ Ability to learn a controlled, longer exhalation, which enables one to use the power of the exhalation to relax the body and calm the mind.
- ✓ Strengthens the diaphragm, but also teaches it to relax, thereby reducing anxiety and tension.
- ✓ Calm, focused mind.
- ✓ Steadying near beginning of the yoga sequence.

Related Yoga Poses
Sukkhasana, Siddhasana, Padmasana, Mula Bandha, Uddiyana Bandha.

HANDS TO WALL BACK STRETCH
– *Ardha Uttanasana*
Ref.: PROGRESSIVE No. 4

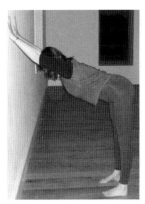

How to Perform the Pose
Stand facing a wall and place your hands on the wall at approximately chest height. On an exhalation, walk your feet back until your back is straight and your feet are parallel and underneath your hips. Hold for up to 30 seconds. To exit, lift the head on an exhalation and walk forwards to stand upright.

Observations
- ▦ Try turning the feet in a little to broaden the back of the pelvis.
- ▦ Make the legs strong: lift the arches of the feet and lift the kneecaps.
- ▦ Feel the stretch on the backs of the legs.
- ▦ Take the tailbone away from the wall (not down or up).
- ▦ Feel length on the front and sides of the trunk.

- Stretch the armpits.
- Take the outer armpits down and allow the chest to float.
- Take the shoulder blades and trapezius muscles down the back.
- Have comfort in the neck with the head in line with the spine.
- Elbows straight and fingers evenly spread.

Variations
- Cup the fingers and place them on the wall rather than flat palms.
- Lift the head to encourage the upper back to move in.
- Lift the sit-bones to encourage the lower back to become less rounded.
- Take the hands higher up the wall.
- Take the hands lower down the wall.
- Take the hands onto a ledge.

Benefits
- ✓ Elongates and stretches the trunk and spine.
- ✓ Stretches the hamstring muscles (back of thighs).
- ✓ Brings mobility to the shoulders and upper back.
- ✓ Enlivens the brain.
- ✓ Stretches the forearms, wrists and hands.

Related Yoga Poses
Uttanasana, Parsvottanasana, Virabhadrasana III.

LYING PELVIC TILTS – *Supta Tadasana*
Ref.: CORE No. 5

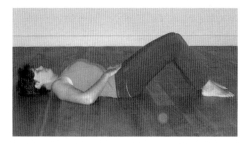

How to Perform the Pose
Lie on your back (supine) and bend your knees to place your feet on the floor, with feet parallel and hip distance apart, and with roughly a 90 degrees angle at the knees. Place your hands on your abdomen.

– ACTIVE (USE ABDOMINAL AND BUTTOCK MUSCLES)
Ref.: CORE 5i

How to Perform the Pose
On an exhalation, engage your abdominal and buttock muscles to perform a tilting of the pelvis that takes your lower back slowly and gently towards the floor: your pubic bone will move up towards your head and the tailbone will move away towards your heels. On an inhalation relax back to a relaxed neutral position. Learn the correct postural position for your pelvis. Repeat x 3.

– PASSIVE (USE LEG MUSCLES)
Ref.: CORE 5ii

How to Perform the Pose
On an exhalation, keeping your feet in place, aim to push your feet away by engaging your leg muscles to effect a slow pelvic tilt with the lower back coming closer to the floor. On the inhalation, keeping your feet still in place, aim to pull your feet towards you to effect a neutral pelvic position. Repeat x 3.

Observations
- The hands will notice that the abdomen feels closer to the spine on the exhalation.
- Not everyone finds this easy, especially the Passive version, so please ask your teacher for help.
- Do not force this action, rather make it slow, comfortable and subtle.
- Do not allow the chest to sink; keep it lifted and open.

Variations
- Arms by the sides, palms up.

Benefits
✓ Pelvic postural re-education ('core' strength, maintenance of pelvic rhythm).
✓ Mobility of lower back.
✓ Strengthening of abdominals, gluteals (buttocks) and leg muscles.

✓ The passive version is very useful if the lower back is strained or tender.
✓ Teaches isolation of different muscle groups.

Related Yoga Poses
Mula Bandha, Ardha Navasana, Uddiyana Bandha.

ABDOMINAL CURL-UPS – *Ardha Navasana Variation*
Refs.: CORE No. 5iii PROGRESSIVE No. 7i (See Next Photograph)

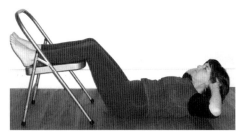

How to Perform the Pose
Lie on your back and on an exhalation place your calves and feet on a chair-seat, so that your knees form an approximate right angle. Spread your fingers as if you are about to pick up two large grapefruits and hold the sides of your head with your fingers. On an exhalation, pull up the pelvic floor muscles, firm your abdomen and using your abdominal muscles, lift your head and shoulders a little way off the floor. On the next inhalation, slowly lower yourself back down to the floor. Repeat x 3.

Observations
■ Imagine the abdomen becoming slimmer at the beginning of the exhalation, as if trying to fit on a pair of tight jeans and then zipping them up from pubis to navel.
■ Use the abdominal muscles and not the throat, neck and arms to lift. No neck tension should be felt after performing – if a little tension is felt, let the head roll gently an inch or two to the right and then to the left and watch the technique next time.
■ The abdomen should not bloat up towards the ceiling – this often happens when lifting too high.
■ Strengthen the abdominal muscles in long, medium and short lengths by lifting slowly and smoothly.
■ Lift up evenly, avoiding the common tendency for one side to be stronger than the other.

Variations

- An imaginary abdominal curl-up can teach more quality of execution than a real one. Try one imaginary one, followed by a real one.
- If stiff in the upper back, start with a book under the head to bring the chin level with the forehead.

ABDOMINAL CURL-UPS BOAT POSE
– *Ardha Navasana Variation*
Ref.: PROGRESSIVE No. 7i

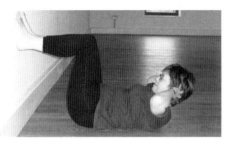

How to Perform the Pose
Box your legs to the wall, by placing your feet on the wall, approximately hip distance apart, with your knees above your hips and your lower legs parallel to the floor. Lift your head and shoulders as in CORE 5iii.

Observations
As previous variation.

Variations

- Tiptoe on the wall, by lifting the heels off when lifting the head up (this will engage the lower abdominals more).
- Squeeze the knees together or into a book placed between the knees when lifting the head up (this will bring more awareness to the central line of the abdomen – useful for split abdominal recti muscles).
- Use the fingers of crossed hands to firmly pull the two sides of the abdomen together in the centre at the level of the navel, when lifting the head up (essential for split abdominal recti muscles).
- Have the legs straight along the floor, pelvic tilt and then lift the head up (may be most useful version for disc problems).
- Lift up diagonally to engage the abdominal oblique muscles, without twisting too much.

■ Push one hand onto the opposite front of thigh near the knee on an exhalation and isometrically resist with the thigh to engage the oblique muscles x 2 to each side (useful for asymmetric sports, e.g. golf or tennis). N.B. in this variation, one foot comes off the wall but the head stays on the floor.

Benefits

✓ Strengthens the abdominals (rectus, obliques and transversus), thereby providing abdominal girdle support for the lumbar spine at the front.
✓ Shoring up the structures of the back by increased abdominal tone.
✓ Additional pelvic and abdominal area strength aids stability in everyday functions, e.g. leaning over the sink or lifting.
✓ Alleviates bloating of abdomen.
✓ Encourages correct functioning of abdominal organs, e.g. bowel, stomach.

Related Yoga Poses

Paripoorna Navasana.

LYING SINGLE LEG RAISES – *Urdhva Prasarita Padasana* Variation
Ref.: PROGRESSIVE No. 7ii

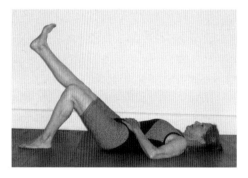

How to Perform the Pose

Lie on your back with your knees bent at a right angle. Place your hands on your abdomen. Straighten your right leg along the floor and have your foot active with your toes above the heel and your leg muscles active. On an exhalation, take your right leg up to 30 degrees and inhale there; on the next exhalation, take your leg up to 60 degrees and inhale there; on the next exhalation, take your leg up to 80 degrees; on an exhalation, keeping your leg strong and active, slowly bring your leg down. Bring your right leg to join your bent left leg and rest for a few moments. Repeat as above with your left leg. Repeat once or twice.

Observations

- Keep the toes spread on the moving leg and aim to hug the leg bones with the leg muscles for strength and support.
- The hands on the lower abdomen should observe the controlling strength of the abdominal and iliopsoas muscles.
- **The abdomen should not bloat or move upwards towards the hands, but should remain firm and steady throughout (important).**
- Do not allow the straight leg to turn out even a little; as the leg reaches the floor, the inner heel skin should touch at the same time as the outer heel skin.
- This is not a hamstring stretch, so do not seek to lift the leg too high or hold at the top; 80 degrees is often further away than one thinks.
- The lower the leg, the harder the muscles have to work to maintain the position, so leave out the lower position(s) if there is difficulty.

Variations

- If the abdominal muscles or back feel too weak to bring the leg down, bend the leg and hug it into the chest using the arms.
- If the abdominal muscles and hip flexors are weak, an easier version is to take the leg up to 80 degrees without stopping and then lower the leg down.
- When stronger, this may be attempted with the other leg straight too.

Benefits

- ✓ Strengthens the abdominal muscles.
- ✓ Strengthens the iliopsoas muscles.
- ✓ Tones the legs.
- ✓ Brings a feeling of general strength and control.

Related Yoga Poses

Paripoorna Navasana, Ardha Navasana.

SEATED CHAIR TWIST – *Bharadvajasana Variation*
Ref.: PROGRESSIVE No. 5i

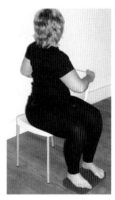

How to Perform the Pose
Sit side on in a firm chair with your right thigh a few inches away from the chair-back. Have your feet hip distance apart, with your feet flat on the floor, parallel and under your knees. Root your tailbone into the chair-seat and lift the spine and chest up. Hold the chair-back with your hands at a comfortable place for you. On an inhalation, lift up and on an exhalation gently turn the ribcage (turn from above the navel only) towards the chair-back, using your hands on the chair to stabilise the position. On each inhalation lift up and on each exhalation relax. Hold comfortably for up to 10–15 seconds. Exit the pose on an exhalation. Turn around on the chair to repeat on your left side. Repeat each side twice. The chair needs to have a flat and level seat – pad it with blankets to correct it if necessary.

Observations
- If the heels do not reach the floor, place a book/block under them (as photo).
- Place the back of the hand in the back of the waist to be sure of the natural curve that should be present, but not exaggerated.
- Make sure the shoulders and back are comfortable with the position of the hands and take the hands lower down the chair-back if necessary.
- Have the elbows a little lifted to the sides, without raising the shoulders, in order to maintain lift and space at the side rib area.
- Aim to turn from the waist upwards, turning the ribcage, chest and shoulders, but not asking the lumbar to turn.
- Take care not to overdo; do with awareness of comfort of all the parts of the trunk.
- Maintain even weight on both buttocks and thighs.
- Keep the shoulders level and relaxed down.
- Maintain an even length to both sides of the trunk.
- Lift the lower abdomen and navel lightly in and up.

▦ Have the head above the tailbone and turn from the heart.

▦ Use the hands to stabilise the pose, but not to pull into the twist.

Variations

- **If stiff in rotational movements, start sitting off-centre facing slightly towards the chair-back**.
- Have a yoga brick, block or wide book between the knees to maintain pelvic alignment broadness.
- Turn from the lower back, to the middle back, to the upper back, to the shoulders and up into the neck with no strain.
- Use the hands, pushing and pulling on the chair-back, to intensify the turn: for stronger, stiffer persons.
- Stretch the arms overhead first to create height on the sides of the body.
- Have a firm bolster to lean into between the chair-back and the trunk (for tender back muscles).

Benefits

- ✓ Mobility in the thoracic area: spine, ribs and upper back.
- ✓ Release of tension in the trunk.
- ✓ Benefits the nervous system; calms jittery nerves and creates healthy nerve exit spaces.
- ✓ Stimulates the mind (the yogic alternative to caffeine).
- ✓ Encourages healthy disc walls.
- ✓ Teaches awareness of movement.
- ✓ Brings clarity and 'get up and go' to the mind.
- ✓ Prevention of headaches.
- ✓ Brings health and circulation to the tissues around the facet joints and encourages synovial fluid within the joints.
- ✓ Detoxing – stimulates the liver, kidneys and intestines.
- ✓ Stimulates the pancreas.

Related Yoga Poses

Parsva Virasana, Utthita Marichyasana III.

STANDING CHAIR TWIST – *Utthita Marichyasana*
Ref.: PROGRESSIVE No. 5ii

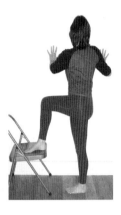

How to Perform the Pose

Place a chair next to an empty wall with the chair touching the wall. Stand side on to the wall, your right thigh approximately 1 foot away from the wall and with the chair in front of you. Stand in Mountain Pose and on an exhalation, place your right foot flat onto the chair-seat (this is **the foot closest to the wall**). Keeping the weight in your standing leg's heel, lift up from that heel towards the top of your head on an inhalation. With your arms hanging down by your sides, on an exhalation begin to turn towards the wall, turning from the bottom of the spine to the middle to the top. When you are facing the wall, place your palms on the wall with the elbows bent. Hold for 10–15 seconds. On each inhalation lift up and on each exhalation relax. To exit the pose, turn back out of the twist on an exhalation, take your foot off the chair and stand in Mountain Pose for a few moments. Move to the other side of the chair and repeat with the other leg up and turning to the left. Repeat a second time to each side with your standing leg heel raised up on a block or book to enable more lumbar lift and, when turned, place your opposite hand on the bent knee to stabilise the knee (see below).

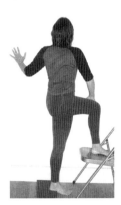

STANDING CHAIR TWIST (Second Variation) (HEEL UP AND HAND TO KNEE) – *Utthita Marichyasana*

Observations

- Stand squarely side on to the wall and keep the standing foot facing directly towards the chair.
- Note that it is the foot of the leg closest to the wall that goes up onto the chair.
- Keep the weight back into the heel of the standing leg to avoid slanting that leg, i.e. keep it perpendicular to the floor (vertical).
- Keep both sides of the body equally long.
- Turn like a spiral from the lowest lumbar vertebra (not much there as it is joined to an immobile sacral segment) and on up to the base of the neck.
- Engage all the small muscles of the back in turn to produce a rotation with awareness.
- Do not lean to one side.
- Keep the shoulders level.
- Relax the jaw, shoulders and neck.
- **Do not overturn or hold too long; make sure the back is comfortable**.
- Avoid leaning the standing leg towards the chair.
- In the second variation, still keep the weight back into the standing heel and lift up from there; notice how it is easier to create a greater lift in the lumbar spine; notice how stabilising the knee gives greater stability at the pelvis and allows more stretch at the outer hip.
- Keep the outer hip in.
- Feel the direction of the bent leg groin moving back into itself (towards the pelvis) for further refining of the alignment of the pose and for more lumbar lift.

Variations

- For extra stability and balance place the front of the chair-seat next to the wall and hold the chair-back and wall as you place your foot up onto the chair.
- If stiff in rotational movements, stand slightly off-centre toward the wall.
- If balance is good, try this in the middle of the room, placing one hand on the opposite bent knee and the other on the back waist in the finished pose.
- Try a version of this lying on the back on the floor, placing one foot onto the knee and crossing the knee over towards the floor (no lower than 1 foot from the floor) to encourage upper lumbar mobility (Crocodile Twist).

■ Place a firm bolster up on end on the thigh and, after turning, lean into the bolster as it rests on the wall (for tense, tender muscles and to prevent backbending or overturning in the lumbar spine).

Benefits
✓ Builds integral strength to the smaller rotational muscles of the spine.
✓ Teaches awareness of correct movement.
✓ Releases tension in the trunk, shoulders and neck (wringing out).
✓ Brings health and circulatory benefits to the facet joints and the disc walls.
✓ Stimulating and invigorating for the brain.
✓ Focusing for the mind.
✓ Detoxing.
✓ Brings greater mobility to the ribcage and diaphragm, enabling healthier breathing leading to better brain function and less anxiety.

Related Yoga Poses
Marichyasana III, Chair Bharadvajasana, Parivrtta Trikonasana.

FRONTAL BODY STRETCH – *Supta Baddhahastasana*
Refs.: CORE No. 6 PROGRESSIVE No. 8

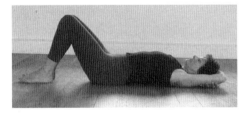

How to Perform the Pose
Lie on your back (supine), with your knees bent and your feet parallel, hip distance apart and flat on the floor. Fold your arms in front of your face, keeping your elbows shoulder distance apart and holding your upper arms above the elbows. On an exhalation, take your folded arms overhead towards the floor over your head. Remain in the pose, breathing steadily for up to 1 minute. To exit the pose: on an exhalation, bring your arms back down. Change the fold of your arms, with the other arm caught first, and repeat the pose.

Observations
■ Check that the body is in a straight line and square with the room.
■ Make sure that the neck is comfortable and long; lift the chin a little and take the shoulder blades and trapezius muscles down the back.

- Stretch the armpits towards the elbows.
- Feel the space on the sides and front of the body.

Variations

- If the shoulders are very stiff and/or painful either (1). place the forearms and wrists onto a support, e.g. a pile of books on the floor above your head or (2). take the arms in and out of the pose whenever necessary.

FRONTAL BODY STRETCH (LEGS STRAIGHT)
– *Supta Tadasana and Baddhahastasana*
Ref.: PROGRESSIVE No. 8 (If Comfortable)

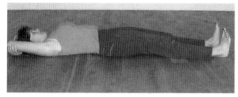

How to Perform the Pose

As you get more practiced at this (after week 7 of the course), **try taking your feet 2 inches further away from you** and wait and observe; then try moving the feet another 2 inches further away from you, observing how different parts of the trunk and spine are involved and enlivened. Try taking your legs out straight along the floor with the feet hip distance apart and push your heels away, as long as this is comfortable for your back.

Benefits

✓ Space at the front of the spine, i.e. for the health of the discs (especially as the pose takes place in the horizontal position), loosens stiff ligaments and muscles at the sides of the spine, thereby benefiting the facet joint and nerve exit spaces.

✓ Lengthens the abdominal and iliopsoas muscles, encouraging long, toned, even muscles.

✓ Beneficial space for chest, abdominal and pelvic organs, leading to enhanced function and health.

✓ Stretches the inter-costal muscles for better breathing.

✓ Lifts the mood and may boost the immune system.

✓ Brings confidence and positivity.

Related Yoga Poses

Sethu Bandhasana with cross bolsters, Urdhva Dhanurasana.

FORWARD STRETCH OVER ONE LEG
– *Parsvottanasana Variation*
Ref.: PROGRESSIVE No. 6i

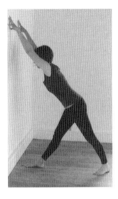

How to Perform the Pose

Stand facing a wall with your right toes approximately 4–12 inches away from the wall and the left foot about 3 feet behind with the left toes turned slightly out. Place your hands on your hips and have the pelvis facing squarely towards the wall. Reach your arms up overhead, stretch up on an inhalation and on an exhalation take your hands forwards and high up on the wall whilst at the same time taking your hips back out into the middle of the room, creating an elongation of the trunk and spine.

Have your fingertips on the wall and hold the pose for up to 20 seconds. To exit the pose: on an exhalation, lift your head and chest up, bring your pelvis towards the wall and step your feet together. Stand with your feet together in Mountain Pose for a few moments, before repeating the pose on the other side with the left foot forwards.

Observations

- It is not easy to keep the pelvis level, so start with the hips facing squarely to the wall and encourage the front leg's side of the hip to move backwards and the back leg's side of the hip to move forwards towards the wall. Ask someone to check and adjust slowly.
- Keep the legs strong and straight throughout.
- Be light on the hands.
- Take the outer armpit down to prevent the chest sagging down.
- Have the head in line with the spine and arms.
- Take the shoulder blades and trapezius muscles down the back and keep the neck comfortable.
- Observe the two-way stretch: the arms going forwards and up and the pelvis and hips going backwards.
- Take the tailbone toward the middle of the room.
- Have the front of the body long.
- Have the back straight and level from hips to shoulders.

■ Keep the inner edge of the front foot and the big toe on the floor.
■ Keep the heel of the back foot down.

Variations
■ Turn the back foot out a little more if the calf stretch is too great or bring the legs closer.
■ Bring the legs closer if the pelvis cannot be level or square.
■ Take the hands underneath the shoulders onto a chair-seat: front foot under the chair; head up, back straight.
■ Take the feet further away from the wall to allow the trunk to be parallel to the floor (if flexible and well-practiced).

Benefits
✓ Stretches the Achilles tendon and the calf muscles.
✓ Stretches the hamstrings.
✓ Strengthens and tones the legs.
✓ Offloads and brings comfort to the back at the sacroiliac joints, facets and nerves.
✓ Brings attention to where the body is in space.
✓ Energises the mind.
✓ Elevation of mood.
✓ Flexibility to the shoulders and upper trunk.

Related Yoga Pose
Ardha Uttanasana.

IMAGINARY CHAIR POSE (BACK TO WALL)
– *Utkatasana Variation*
Ref.: PROGRESSIVE No. 6ii

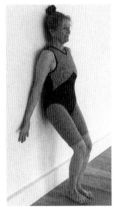

How to Perform the Pose

Stand in Mountain Pose (upright) with your feet together and your heels approximately 9 inches away from the wall. With your hands on the wall, lean back to rest your pelvis and trunk on the wall. On an exhalation, bend your knees, keeping your heels down. Place your hands on your abdomen and take the back of the waist down the wall and the abdomen in towards the wall and up. Either place your hands on your hips or place the backs of your hands on the wall, maintaining the position of the abdomen and the lift of the chest. Hold for up to 20 seconds. To exit the pose, press the fingers into the wall, straighten the legs and stand upright.

Observations

▪ Have the weight in the heels and lift the shins up; try lifting the toes to learn this.

▪ Be even on the feet: both right and left and inner and outer feet.

▪ Take the inner groins down.

▪ Take the tailbone and back of the waist down.

▪ Allow the outer thighs to move forwards toward the middle of the room.

▪ Note the similarities to Eagle Pose.

▪ Observe how the abdomen wants to spill into the room, the pelvis may want to tilt forwards and the lower back may wish to move strongly away from the wall; aim to resist all these tendencies.

▪ Lift the chest up and spread the collarbones to the sides.

▪ Lengthen the back of the neck and do not force the head to go back to the wall; having the head an inch or so from the wall is fine.

▪ Observe how placing the backs of the hands on the wall and having the palms facing forwards encourages a broadening, opening feeling for the chest.

Variations

- Take the arms up overhead without strain (when strong).
- Do without the support of the wall, keeping the trunk upright.
- Relate this to lying on the back with knees slightly bent.
- Take the feet further from the wall and take the trunk lower down the wall, to strengthen the quadriceps muscles more.
- Have the feet a little apart and keep the weight even on all 4 corners of the feet with the knees neither falling in nor out (teaches correct knee alignment).

Benefits

- ✓ Teaches awareness for postural re-education in the upright position.
- ✓ Lessens excessive lumbar lordosis (sway back).
- ✓ Uses the support of the wall for alignment.
- ✓ Teaches broadening of the back of the pelvis.
- ✓ Lift of the chest, without overarching the lumbar spine: teaches spinal curve links.
- ✓ Strengthens the legs.

Related Yoga Poses

Garudasana, Tadasana.

SINGLE LEG LOCK – *Supta Padangustasana Variation*
Refs.: CORE No. 7 PROGRESSIVE No. 9i

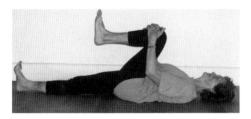

How to Perform the Pose

Lie on your back with both knees bent and feet flat on the floor. On an exhalation bring your right leg towards the chest; on another exhalation take your left leg straight along the floor with the toes above the heel. Hold your right leg over the shin by interlocking your fingers. Hold this position, breathing steadily for up to 60 seconds. To exit the pose, bring your straight leg back to bent on an exhalation and place the bent leg back on the floor to join it. Repeat with the left leg held to your chest. After this come back to symmetry by holding both legs gently into the chest for 10–15 seconds. (**If you feel unstable at the back of the pelvis**, as is sometimes the case when menstruating for instance, **try clenching the buttock muscles in this position before you move**.)

Observations

- Observe space in the trunk at the front (on the straight leg side) and at the back (on the bent leg side).
- Avoid tension at the front of the groin by allowing the leg to come in slowly and softly and do not grip the leg in too tightly.
- Try keeping the bent leg foot and leg very relaxed and the straight leg foot and leg very active: observe the contrast.
- Sometimes keep both feet active with toes above the heels and observe more awareness deep within the hip-joint.
- Resist the tendency to allow the straight leg to roll out by taking the inner groin and inner knee towards the floor.
- Stretch the inner heel of the straight leg away.
- Imagine pressing the straight leg foot away into an imaginary wall.
- Relax the arms, shoulders, neck and throat.
- Relax the facial muscles, especially the mouth and jaw.

Variations

- **Begin with both legs straight and then bring one leg into the chest (= PROGRESSIVE 9i).**
- Work with the breath, by gently bringing the knee closer in towards the chest on the exhalation and then away by straightening the arms on the inhalation.
- Hold the hands at the back of the thigh if the hip and/or knee is stiff (observe the beneficial space this gives to the back of the knee during this weightless knee bend).
- Hold a belt around the back of the thigh, if the arms seem too short.
- With both legs straight along the floor, place both feet flat on a wall; keeping the sole of one foot pressed into the skirting board of the wall, bring one knee into the chest (better action of the straight leg).
- Give the hip and lumbar traction by placing a long looped belt from the top of the bent leg groin to the straight leg foot (this previously straight leg should now become slightly bent). To gain traction (and possible sacroiliac correction) bring the knee in and then away from the chest keeping the tension on the belt).

SINGLE LEG LOCK WITH HEAD LIFT
– *Supta Padangustasana Variation*
Ref.: PROGRESSIVE 9ii

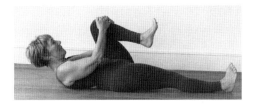

How to Perform the Pose

Prepare as previous pose. (This may not suit you if you have neck problems – in this case, you can do this in your mind instead as an imaginary lift, engaging the abdominal muscles.) Draw your abdomen back towards your spine and, on an exhalation and without pulling with your arms, lift your head and shoulders into an Abdominal Curl-Up. Keep the back of your neck long and your jaw and tongue relaxed. Lower on your inhalation.

Benefits

- ✓ Gently stretches the paraspinal muscles on the bent leg side and the hip flexors on the straight leg side.
- ✓ Gives gentle traction to the lumbar spine, with the straight leg lengthening action.
- ✓ Lessens lumbar curve.
- ✓ Lengthens and balances iliopsoas muscles.
- ✓ PROGRESSIVE 9ii opens up the facet joints on the bent leg side, especially benefiting the lowest L5–S1 joints. This can give great pain relief at that area.
- ✓ Can be corrective for sacroiliac problems.
- ✓ Stretches the hip flexors.
- ✓ Allows a longer more even stride when walking.

Related Yoga Poses

Utthita Hasta Padangustasana, Ardha Navasana.

SINGLE LEG LOCK TO HAMSTRING STRETCH
– *Supta Padangustasana*
Ref.: PROGRESSIVE No. 7iii

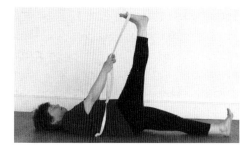

How to Perform the Pose
Lie on your back and bend your right leg gently in towards your chest. Place a long belt on the ball of your foot. Holding the belt in both hands, on an exhalation straighten your leg up towards the ceiling. Hold the pose for up to 30 seconds. To exit the pose, bring your knee back down towards your chest, straighten your leg out along the floor and rest for a few moments. Repeat with your left leg.

Observations

- The raised leg knee should be straight; it should be straight at the back of the knee as well as at the front of the knee.
- Feel the stretch on the back of the raised leg and use the power of the exhalations to lessen the sensation for relief and for relaxing of the muscles.
- Do not be aggressive in this pose.
- Aim to be firm on the front of the leg.
- Keep space and length at the side of the raised leg waist; move the outer hip away with the thumb.
- Relax the arms, shoulders and neck.
- Keep the back of the neck long.
- Relax the facial muscles, especially the eyes and mouth.
- Spread the toes of both feet.
- Take the thigh-bones from front to back on both legs.
- Stretch from the inner groin to the inner heel on the lower leg.
- Take the inner knee and inner thigh down on the lower leg and keep the toes above the heel with an active foot.
- Lift the chest and heart up towards the ceiling and towards the face in order not to jam the lumbar into the floor.
- **Keep a natural curve at the lumbar spine; do not bring the leg in too close, but use more belt length.**

Variations

- Place a folded towel at the back of the waist to maintain the lumbar curve (especially for disc problems).
- Have the lower leg foot pressing into a wall.
- Put the lower leg heel up on a block or a book.
- Take the leg up and then turn the thigh-bone in its hip socket to take the leg out to the side, holding the belt in one hand (relaxes the piriformis and stretches the adductor muscles).
- Take the leg up and then across the body about 6 inches (stretches the piriformis and the abductor muscles).

Benefits

- ✓ Stretches the hamstrings.
- ✓ Teaches one to learn the power of the exhalation to relieve pain.
- ✓ Relieving for, and preventative of, arthritic hips and knees.
- ✓ Relieves any swelling in the legs (oedema, varicose veins, arthritic knees).
- ✓ Antidote to stress.
- ✓ Stretches the sciatic nerve.
- ✓ Improves walking stride.
- ✓ Tones the legs.

Related Yoga Poses

Utthita Hasta Padangustasana, Utthita Trikonasana (side variation).

ALL FOURS – *Chaturangasana*
Ref.: CORE No. 8 What To Do If... No. 3d

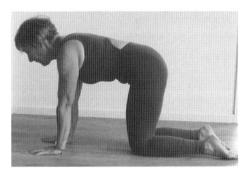

How to Perform the Pose

Kneel on the floor with your knees under your hips and your hands just in front of your shoulders. Hold still for up to 60 seconds. You may like to gently, steadily and smoothly rock forwards and back.

Observations

▨ Have level padding under the knees, e.g. a folded blanket, but have the hands on the firm floor for knee and wrist comfort.

▨ Notice how comfortable the back feels in this four-legged position.

▨ Have the head in line with the spine, neither dropped nor held up too high; look at the floor by the fingertips.

▨ Spread the fingers evenly and press all the knuckles down whilst stretching the fingers straight.

▨ Firm the arms from the floor up into the shoulders.

▨ Feel a firmness at the armpit area.

▨ Find a neutral position for the back: no humped back and no sagging abdomen.

▨ Feel the top of the head aiming directly forwards (not down) and the tailbone aiming directly backwards (not up).

▨ Whilst rocking forwards and back, feel the body and mind being soothed like a baby being rocked.

▨ Whilst rocking, observe the involvement of all the different joints: wrists, shoulders, spinal joints, hips, knees.

Variations

ALL FOURS OVER CHAIR (STILL – NO ROCKING)

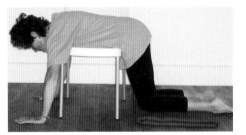

■ This can be performed over a chair-seat giving abdominal support and more rest to the back muscles. The seat of the chair must be flat (pad with a blanket if it is not) and your knees must be solidly on the floor or support of a block or firm blanket (i.e. it must not feel as if your knees are 'floating'. (Ref.: What To Do If… 3.d photo above).

■ Move back into Pose of the Child (**Ref.:** CORE 9) and stay for a few seconds.

■ Arch the back up with chin in to chest and tailbone in on an exhalation and come back to neutral on an inhalation.

■ Pull up the navel towards the spine on an exhalation to strengthen and engage the deep transverse abdominal muscles.

■ Leg lifts: take the toes of one straight leg to the floor behind; keeping the abdomen in and the pelvis on that side down, lift the leg a little (similar to prone single leg lifts, but more '**core stability**' needed here – check the lumbar curve does not increase and hips should be level, so aim for quality movement rather than a high lift). Hold for 5–10 seconds.

■ Arm lifts: take the fingertips of one straight arm to the floor in front; keeping the abdomen in and with no strain in the neck, lift the arm and stretch it forwards. Hold for 5–10 seconds.

Benefits

✓ Offloads the structures of the back and allows the back muscles to rest.
✓ Teaches the correct lumbar curve.
✓ Pain-relieving position.
✓ Rocking allows the brain to lose its grip and worries, thereby allowing the muscles to release and relax.
✓ Gentle lubrication of joints through the movement of rocking, each vertebral segment encouraged to be involved as in a well-oiled bicycle chain – especially good to move in this way in inflammatory conditions.

Related Poses

Adho Mukha Svanasana, Adho Mukha Virasana.

POSE OF THE CHILD – FOLDED ARMS TO CHAIR – *Adho Mukha Virasana* Variation
Ref.: CORE No. 9i

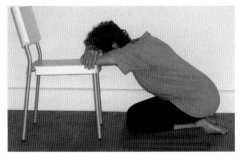

How to Perform the Pose

Sit to your heels in a kneeling position, with your knees slightly apart, using supports as necessary. On an exhalation, bend forwards from your hips, keeping your back straight and maintaining the length on the front of your body to place your elbows on a chair-seat in front of you. Rest your forehead on the palms of your hands for a few moments. If comfortable to do so, fold your arms and rest them onto the chair-seat and stretch forwards a little more to rest your forehead on your forearms. Hold for up to 1 minute. To exit the pose, keep your back muscles relaxed, by using your arms to come up. Change the fold of your arms halfway through or come up and go back in.

Observations

- For sciatica or leg symptoms from disc problems, read Observations in the following pose and it may be advisable to leave out this pose.
- When entering the pose, place the fingers at the top of the thighs to ensure that the bend occurs at the hips and not at the waist.
- Keep length on the front of the body, when entering the pose by keeping length from pubis to navel, navel to front ribs and by lifting the chest forwards.
- Have the elbows shoulder distance apart in order to feel an armpit stretch and to prevent collapsing of the chest.
- Hold the upper arms near the elbows with the opposite hands in order to keep the elbows shoulder distance apart and to provide stability to the shoulder girdle.
- Encourage the shoulder blades and trapezius muscles to move down the back, so as not to crowd out the neck.
- Have a comfortable length at the back of the neck: no wrinkles at the back of the neck.
- Encourage the forehead skin to move downwards from the hairline to the eyebrows, thereby relaxing the forehead muscles and calming the brain.

Variations

- Have a 1 inch thick, evenly folded blanket at the back of the knees for stiffness in the knees and also one or two books/blocks or cushions under the buttocks on top of the heels until total comfort at the knees is felt.
- **Chair-seated forward bend (CORE No. 1) is a good alternative that does not involve the knees**.
- Place a rolled blanket under the front of the ankles, if they are stiff and the feet are painful or cramp occurs.

Benefits

- ✓ Gives confidence to bend forwards with support.
- ✓ Calming for the brain.
- ✓ Releases tension in the shoulders.
- ✓ Relaxes the lower back muscles.

✓ Stretches the tops of the feet and front ankles.
✓ Relieves headaches.

POSE OF THE CHILD – *Adho Mukha Virasana*
Refs.: CORE No. 9ii PROGRESSIVE No.10

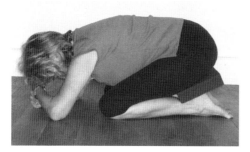

How to Perform the Pose
Sit on the floor in a kneeling position with your knees slightly apart. If on a hard floor, always use an evenly folded blanket under your knees and ankles. On an exhalation, bend forwards from your hips, keeping the front of your body long and your hips comfortably down, to place your forehead on your stacked fists resting on the floor, with elbows bent. You must be comfortable and not have any leg pain or symptoms – if you experience these, exit the pose and spend extra time lying on your abdomen. Stay at two-fist height or, if comfortable, lower on an exhalation to one-fist height or even to rest your forehead on the floor. Hold for up to 2 minutes. Exit the pose on an exhalation, by pressing your hands into the floor in front of your knees and using your arm muscles to lift your body up with your back muscles remaining relaxed. Inhale once upright.

Observations
◼ **Never feel leg symptoms (pain, pins and needles or numbness) in this or the previous chair version of this pose. Where there is a current disc problem, if there is too much of a downward bend rather than a forward bend with length on the front body, this position can prevent the disc healing, so leave it out if it gives you leg symptoms during or after or if you have these symptoms in any case and ask for advice. You may be advised to substitute Table-Top Back Relaxer (CORE 1 with the legs back and straight) instead.** This will be relevant for most forward bends.

◼ Use a long exhalation to enter the pose.

◼ When entering the pose, place the fingers at the top of the thighs to ensure that the bend occurs at the hips and not at the waist.

◼ Keep length at the front of the body, when entering the pose by keeping length from pubis to navel, navel to front ribs and by lifting the chest forwards.

■ Feel a comfortable stretch sensation on the muscles of the lower back; if too much stretch is felt, bring the head higher or come back to the chair (CORE 9i).

■ Encourage the shoulder blades and trapezius muscles to move down the back, so as not to crowd out the neck.

■ Have a comfortable length at the back of the neck: no wrinkles at the back of the neck.

■ Encourage the forehead skin to move downwards from the hairline to the eyebrows, thereby relaxing the forehead muscles and calming the brain.

■ Breathe well into the back body to release tension on the exhalations.

Variations

■ If you have a disc problem see the end of this pose description and do PRONE LYING instead of this.

■ Folded arms to chair-seat as in CORE 9i.

■ Have a 1 inch thick, evenly folded blanket at the back of the knees for stiffness in the knees and also one or two books/blocks or cushions under the buttocks on top of the heels until total comfort at the knees is felt.

■ Chair-Seated Forward Bend (Ref.: CORE 1) is a good alternative that does not involve the knees.

■ Table-Top Back Relaxer (Ref.: CORE 1) is a good alternative to relax the back muscles without compromising space for the discs, especially with legs further back and straight.

■ Place a rolled blanket under the front of the ankles, if they are stiff.

■ Place a book/block under the forehead and stretch the arms forward with the palms on the floor, taking the outer armpit downwards.

■ Place a book/block under the buttocks and a couple of books/blocks under the forehead.

■ Lie the front of the body along a firm bolster support (for extra soothing for the abdominal organs and back muscles); feels more like Table-Top Back Relaxer (Ref.: CORE 1).

■ Have the arms by the sides, elbows bent and palms facing up by the feet (extra relaxation at the back of the shoulders).

■ Place the weight of a large book, heavy blanket or a sandbag on any tense areas of the back to encourage deeper muscular relaxation.

Benefits

✓ Gives confidence to bend forwards because of its stable and limiting support.

✓ Calming for the brain.

✓ Releases tension in the shoulders.

✓ Relaxes the back muscles, especially in the lower back.

✓ Stretches the tops of the feet and front ankles.

✓ Opens and calms the facet joints.

✓ Brings stillness to the mind.

✓ Lessens anxiety and brings a feeling of security.

✓ Pain-relieving from muscle spasm pain as long as the stretch sensation is adjusted to optimum, i.e. not too low down with head.

Related Yoga Poses

Paschimottanasana, Uttanasana.

PRONE LYING – *Prone Savasana* – (Alternative to above pose and also to the 3 following front-lying poses)

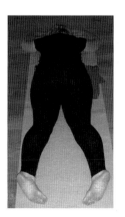

■ **If a disc problem is present, instead of previous pose, lie prone as in the photograph above, and rest on front, possibly with a pillow under whole trunk or under abdomen and pelvis. (Useful to rest prone 3 x a day for at least 5 minutes).**

PRONE SINGLE LEG LIFTS – *Salabhasana (– Ekapada)*
Refs.: CORE No. 10 PROGRESSIVE No. 11i

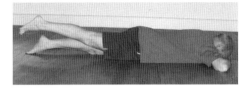

How to Perform the Pose
Lie on the floor on your abdomen (prone). Bend your elbows to the sides and place your forehead on top of your fingertips. Tucking your tailbone in and taking the flesh and muscles of the buttocks towards the heels, on an exhalation lift your right leg a little off the floor. Hold for up to one breath and then lower your leg. Repeat with your left leg x 1 to 3.

Observations
■ Tucking the tailbone in and taking the buttocks towards the heels will give pelvic stability and prevent the leg from lifting too high.
■ Keep both sides of the pelvis on the floor.
■ No strain or pinched feeling should be felt in the lower back area, rather a warm strong feeling to the muscles; so avoid going for height and mobility, rather for firm strength and comfort.
■ If the foot cramps, tuck toes under on the floor and push that heel away.
■ Take the leg up and down slowly and smoothly, rather like an extremely slow swimming front crawl.

Variations
■ If not comfortable lying prone, place a lengthwise pillow under whole trunk (or a crosswise pillow under pelvis and/or abdomen).
■ Try doing the pose with the toes pointed (length to front of the leg and hip); -try doing the pose with the heels stretched away avoiding lifting too high (toes almost on the floor (length to the back of the leg and hip); try doing both these actions together, 'active foot', by pulling the toes back towards you, but at the same time pushing the heel away and the ball of the foot simultaneously – the ball of the foot will be further away than the heel, but not as far away as when foot is pointed.
■ Lift the leg only a millimetre and observe better quality of strength.

Benefits
✓ Strengthens the back of the lower body, including the buttocks and legs.
✓ Brings strength to the back body to encourage loosening of the hip flexors at front of the body.

✓ Strengthens the erector spinae (back) muscles.
✓ Allows a longer, more even stride for walking.

Related Yoga Poses
Bhujangasana, Dhanurasana, Virabhadrasana III.

COBRA POSE – *Bhujangasana*
Ref.: PROGRESSIVE No. 11ii

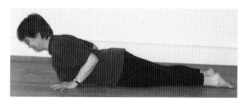

How to Perform the Pose
Lie on your front and place your palms flat on the floor beside your lower ribs, fingers pointing forwards and elbows up. Place your forehead on the floor, tuck your tailbone in and take the buttock muscles down towards the heels with the feet an inch or so apart. On an exhalation curl your chest up off the floor into a low, comfortable backbend. Inhale well once you are in your comfortable pose and keep breathing evenly. Hold the pose for up to 15 seconds. To exit, on an exhalation lower your chest forwards and down. Relax your arms by your sides with palms facing up and turn your head to one side. Rest for a few moments with toes in and heels out (as shown in photo after next).

Observations
■ **Stay within and do not exceed your comfortable easy capacity – keep low**.
■ Stretch the arms overhead along the floor before performing the pose to get more length to the body.
■ Feel the upper back muscles moving into the body.
■ Aim to involve the thoracic spine in the backbend, but do not over-involve the lumbar spine.
■ Look forwards and down (not up) to keep length on the back of the neck.
■ Stretch the legs back to encourage length in the lumbar spine.
■ The emphasis here is on back body strength, not mobility, so do not lift too high.
■ Do not clench the buttock muscles towards the centre, rather move them down towards the heels.

- Pay attention to the sensation at the lowest lumbar area; there should be absolute comfort here.
- Keep the elbows bent by the sides and the shoulders down away from the ears.
- **Never be competitive in yoga**.
- Try the pose with the eyes closed to truly observe how the body is responding (i.e. keep within your comfort limit).
- After performing the pose, place the hands under the abdomen and bring it up towards the front ribs and tuck the tailbone down as well to relieve the back muscles.

Variations

- Like a sphinx: be on the elbows looking under the belly (tailbone in) and look forwards little by little to encourage each thoracic vertebral segment to individually be involved in the back-bending action. Bend the arms out to the sides to lower down and exit the pose.
- Have a pillow under the abdomen and pelvis to lessen the intensity of the backbend.

Benefits

✓ Spinal mobility in extension.
✓ Strength to the back of the body.
✓ Stimulates the cardiovascular system.
✓ Space at the front of the ribs.
✓ Healthy migration of the disc nucleus forwards to prevent posterior herniation.
✓ Encourages circulation to the discs.
✓ Health for the lungs.
✓ Invigoration of the mind.
✓ Increase in energy levels.
✓ Confidence.
✓ Elevated mood – "Light-heartedness".

Related Yoga Poses

Salabhasana, Dhanurasana, Ustrasana.

SACROILIAC STABILISER (SIS)
– Chaturanga Dandasana Variation
Ref.: CORE No. 11 PROGRESSIVE No. 11iii

What To Do If... No. 3e

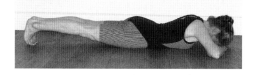

How to Perform the Pose

Lie on the floor on your abdomen (prone), with your elbows bent and your forehead resting on your fingertips. With your feet together and tailbone tucked lightly in, tuck your toes under, as if tiptoeing on the floor. On an exhalation firm your legs, allowing your knees to lift and firm your buttocks. Hold for up to 20 seconds. Repeat once more. Relax well between repetitions with the toes in and heels out.

Observations

- Firm the legs strongly as all the muscles hug against the leg bones.
- Tuck the tailbone in, take the buttock muscles towards the heels and firm the muscles around the sacroiliac joints.
- Feel the symmetry of the pelvis: the floor being the teaching aid.
- Observe the firm, strong feel at the sacrum.
- This pose is hard work: it may make one want to hold the breath but do continue to breathe steadily.
- The relaxation after this SIS pose is as important as the actual active pose.

PRONE LYING – Relaxation Between Repetitions SIS

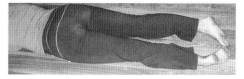

Ref.: CORE No. 11
PROGRESSIVE No. 11iii

What To Do If... No. 3e

- During the relaxation turn the head comfortably to one side, alternating sides, and relax the arms. Relax the legs well, back of the thighs relaxing from inside to out, encouraged by the feet relaxing with the toes in and heels out. Completely relax the buttocks and back of pelvis on the exhalations, by relaxing from the centre to the sides.

Variations and Benefits
See below under PROGRESSIVE Variation.

SACROILIAC STABILISER (SIS) WITH HEAD LIFT
– *Chaturanga Dandasana*
Ref.: PROGRESSIVE No. 11iii

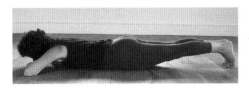

How to Perform the Pose
Perform as in the previous variation of the pose. Lift your head up until your nose is approximately 4 inches from the floor, still looking downwards.

Observations
- If it is not possible to do this without losing the power of the legs and the action of the tailbone tucking in and down, try lifting the head so that the nose is only 1 inch from the floor or keep the head down (CORE 11).
- Feel the warmth and strength on the whole back body (especially useful for strengthening the mid-back area).

Variations
- Place a pillow under trunk (as in previous pose).
- Do not over-tuck the tailbone in cases of flattened lumbar curve.
- Have feet hip distance apart to enable better taking in of the tailbone (as in classical Chaturanga Dandasana pose).

Benefits
- Stabilises the sacroiliac joints; strengthens the back pelvis.
- Brings symmetry to the pelvis.
- Gives great relief (and prevents further backache) if one has overdone forward bends, e.g. gardening; perform this as soon as possible after the offending forward-bending strain.
- Brings strength to the whole of the back body, thereby aiding spinal posture.
- Usefully uses the back body musculature in an active way.
- Teaches awareness of where the piriformis and gluteal muscles are in order to be able to relax them afterwards.

✓ PROGRESSIVE variation strengthens top lumbar/bottom thoracic area (useful if weak or slouched).

Related Yoga Poses
Salabhasana, Urdhva Mukha Svanasana.

LYING TWISTS – CORE Variations –
Jatara Parivartanasana Variation (as *Bharadvajasana*)
Ref.: CORE Nos. 12i, 12ii, 12iii   What To Do If... Nos. 3ii/iii
(For PROGRESSIVE Nos. See Later)

(Have Arms At 45° Only)

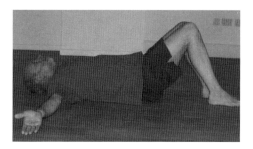

How to Perform the Pose
Lie on your back with your knees bent, your feet flat on the floor and hip distance apart. Take your arms out to the sides at shoulder-height with the palms facing upwards....

– TILT
Ref.: CORE No. 12i   (What To Do If... No. 3fi)

How to Perform the Pose
Allow your knees to tilt a small amount, no more than 4 inches, to the left. Hold for 30 seconds. Bring your knees back to centre on an exhalation and repeat to the right side. You may repeat to each side.

Observations
- The back of the pelvis is completely on the floor.
- This subtle tilt gives a good opportunity to observe subtle reactions within the body.
- Observe the postural readjustments of the iliopsoas muscles that occur deep at the back of the tummy on the two sides: the left slacker side tones up, when the knees are tilted subtly to the left.
- Note that this is the starting point of any twist and will teach where any restrictions are.

– STEADY MOVEMENT IN AND OUT
Ref.: CORE No. 12ii

How to Perform the Pose
(See previous photograph) On an exhalation allow your knees to go down slowly, steadily and comfortably to the left and on the inhalation bring your knees back up. On the next exhalation take your knees to the other side. Move steadily and smoothly synchronising the movement of your legs with your breath x 6–10 breaths.

Observations
- Do not allow the body to go further than is completely comfortable; start with less movement and be attentive to how every part of the body feels.
- Observe how the pelvis does not remain on the floor in this version.
- For the first few breaths, the knees will probably not go down very far, but as the breath naturally lengthens and the body relaxes, the knees are likely to go PROGRESSIVE ly further inch by inch with each breath.
- The breath and the movement of the legs should be equally smooth and steady.
- Feel the control from the abdominals; the knees should not drop, but should move steadily with control.
- The feet will tilt onto their sides when the knees go to the side.

– FEET HIP DISTANCE, HOLD, WITH HEAD TURN –
Jatara Partivartanasana Variation (as *Bharadvajasana*)
Ref.: CORE No. 12iii

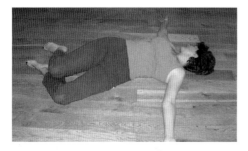

How to Perform the Pose
On an exhalation, allow your knees to go down to the left as far as is comfortable. Should you run out of exhalation, wait at the point your legs have reached to inhale and then lower your knees further on the next exhalation. Once you have gone

down as far as is comfortable, allow your head to roll the opposite way, to the right. Hold for 15–30 seconds. To exit the pose, bring your head back to the centre and bring your knees up on an exhalation. Repeat to the right (knees right and then head left).

Observations

- Be comfortable and do not move quickly or force.
- Be attentive to the comfort of the back and waist areas.
- Allow the legs to come apart as much as necessary; it is best if the bottom leg eventually reaches the ground, but it is not necessary for the top leg to stay with the bottom leg.
- Note the spiralling twist throughout the spine from the lumbar region to the head.
- Feel a gentle stretch across the pectoral chest area; stretch the arms and hands without tension to feel more stretch here.
- Before taking the head to the side, check that the shoulders are away from the ears and that the shoulder blades are moving down the back.
- Do not move the head first in an action, or the awareness within the body will be lessened.
- Should the musculature feel too weak to bring both legs up at once, bring the top leg up first (useful if legs went down too far or pose was held for too long).

Variations

- **Variation** CORE 12iii may be done by placing the knees down onto support (such as a couple of pillows) at the side or with a pillow between the knees.
- Arms may be higher than shoulder-height in order to emphasize the twist higher up the trunk.

Benefits

Variation CORE 12i:

- ✓ Teaches confidence and participation in the necessary contributory muscles and joints for all twisting actions.
- ✓ Having the feet apart provides stability for comfortable movement.
- ✓ Balances the psoas muscles for a balanced pelvis and comfortable sacroiliac joints.

✓ Encourages the stiff parts to move and the weaker hyper-mobile parts to hold back.

✓ Keeps the mind focused, aware and steady.

Variation CORE 12ii:

✓ Lubricates the facet joints by the movement.

✓ Strengthens the back muscles and the abdominals.

✓ Improves 'core stability', allowing for comfortable everyday movements.

✓ Mobilises or maintains mobility of the vertebral segments.

✓ Encourages the body, mind and breath to feel united.

Variation CORE 12iii:

✓ As ii. above, but more stretching and making space for long-term freedom of movement.

All Variations

✓ Stretches and thereby encourages movement and added circulation to the vertebral segments.

✓ When done without strain, encourages health to come to the disc walls.

✓ Encourages health of the nervous system, by freeing up the nerve exit spaces.

✓ Calms or stimulates the nervous system depending on the balancing required to bring harmony to the nerves.

✓ Can relieve irritable bowel syndrome (IBS) and aid digestion (N.B. taking the knees to the left side first in order that the body twists to the right is the most natural way to perform these twisting poses for the digestive system).

✓ Can aid kidney, liver, gall bladder and pancreatic function.

✓ Can lessen respiratory tension or congestion.

✓ Releases tension in the muscles of the trunk and is de-stressing for the brain.

✓ Stimulates (squeezes) and relaxes (makes space for) the organs of the trunk.

✓ Encourages healthy use of the diaphragm and freedom from stiffness at the ribs.

✓ Twists are very beneficial for the health of the back and these twists are all done with the floor as an alignment teacher; doing the twists in the horizontal position acts as a gravitational weight reliever.

✓ Helps define the waist and improve body shape.

✓   Stretches the outer thigh and hip.
✓   Increases energy levels.

Related Yoga Poses
Parivrtta Trikonasana, Bhardvajasana.

LYING TWISTS (Start Position in Photo Below) – PROGRESSIVE Variations – *Jatara Parivartanasana*
Ref.: PROGRESSIVE Nos. 2i, 12ii, 12iii
(CORE Nos. See Before)

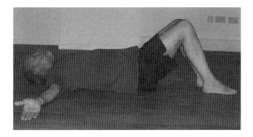

How to Perform the Pose
Lie on your back with your knees bent and place your feet flat on the floor. Take your arms out to the sides at shoulder-height with your palms facing upwards.

– LYING TWISTS (FEET WIDE, ONE KNEE IN) – *Jatara Parivartanasana* Variation (as *Gomukhasana*)
Ref.: PROGRESSIVE No. 12i.a

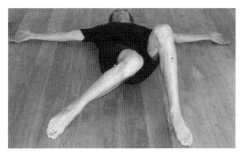

How to Perform the Pose
Take your feet to 2–2½ feet apart. Maintaining the upright position of your left leg, on an exhalation, allow your right leg to roll in and take your right knee slowly, comfortably and gently downwards towards your left ankle. Hold for up to 30 seconds. On an exhalation bring your knee up. Repeat with your left leg.

Observations
▨   Observe tightness or restrictions on the outer hip, thigh or waist areas and lessen these with the exhalations.
▨   Breathe steadily.

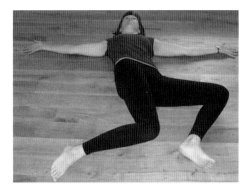

– LYING TWISTS (FEET WIDE, BOTH KNEES DOWN) – *Jatara Parivartanasana* Variation (as *Bharadvajasana*)
Ref.: Progressiive No. 12i.B

Still with your feet 2–2½ feet apart, on an exhalation take both knees slowly and comfortably down to the left. Hold for up to 30 seconds. On an exhalation bring your knees up. Repeat taking the knees down to the right.

Observations
- Notice how there is more space within the front of the trunk.
- Observe how this twist provides more traction to the spine and space for the discs.
- With the legs wider the emphasis of the twist is lower down the spine and towards the outside of the body.
- Enjoy the long line from the right armpit to the right knee and the lengthening of the iliopsoas back and pelvic muscles deep inside the abdomen.

– LYING TWISTS (LEGS CROSSED) – *Jatara Parivartanasana* Variation (as *Ardha Matsyendrasana* and *Garudasana*)
Ref.: PROGRESSIVE No. 12ii:

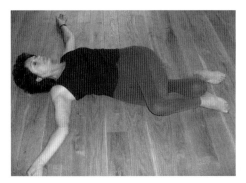

How to Perform the Pose
This can be a strong twist, so go in with care and attentiveness: go slowly, minimally and gently or leave it out.

With your knees bent, bring your feet and knees together. Take your right leg over the left leg to cross your legs with the thighs closed. On an exhalation, slowly take the legs down to the left. Use your left hand to catch the underside of the knees until you feel secure and comfortable. Hold for up to 30 seconds. On an exhalation, bring your knees back upright, using your left hand to aid if necessary. Repeat with the other cross of legs and to the other side.

Observations
◼ Notice how the abdominals and back muscles have to work harder to take the knees into this crossed variation.
◼ Notice the emphasis in this variation is on the outer hip and pelvic areas.

– LYING TWISTS (FEET TOGETHER)
– *Jatara Parivartanasana*
Ref.: PROGRESSIVE No. 12iii

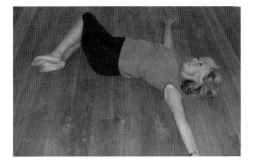

How to Perform the Pose
With your knees bent, bring your feet and knees together. Keeping the inside edges of your feet together, on an exhalation, take your knees slowly down to the left. Allow your knees to come a little apart to prevent asking too much of your back muscles and joints. Keep your right foot stacked onto the side of your left foot. Go as far as is comfortable, aiming to allow your bottom leg to rest on the floor for stability. Hold for up to 30 seconds. On an exhalation bring your legs up to the centre. Repeat to your right side.

Observations
◼ **If necessary, bring one leg up before the other to make leaving the pose easier**.
◼ Notice the emphasis in this variation is on the centre of the body.
◼ More strength is required in this variation.
◼ If this variation brings too much tension or the feet do not want to stack, allow the feet to roll in place on the floor.
◼ Continue to breathe steadily in all these variations.
◼ Observe the inhalation making space and the exhalation relaxing the body.

Variations

- Go back to the CORE Lying Twists if they suit better, as they provide the foundation to move on to these other PROGRESSIVE variations.
- In Variation PROGRESSIVE 12ii – gently rock over the buttock of the top leg before going down in order to massage and warm those muscles.
- In Variation PROGRESSIVE 12iii – Relaxed version: have a bolster between the knees or allow the knees to go down onto a support.
- In Variation PROGRESSIVE 12iii – Easier version: keep the feet on the floor and let the feet roll onto their sides.
- In Variation PROGRESSIVE 12iii – Harder version: keep the knees together and lower as far as is comfortable.

Benefits

Variation PROGRESSIVE 12i.a

✓ Stretches across, and spreads the back of, the sacroiliac area.
✓ Stretches the piriformis and gluteal muscles.

Variation PROGRESSIVE 12i.b

✓ Gives traction to the spine, opening up the facet joints on one side and relieving bulging discs.
✓ Lengthens the iliopsoas muscles.
✓ Provides extra space for the organs of the trunk.

Variation PROGRESSIVE 12ii

✓ Gives a further stretch and spreading to the sacroiliac areas.
✓ Stretches the piriformis muscle, which is deep within the mid buttock.
✓ Piriformis muscle tightness is often contributory to the symptoms of sciatica (pain, pins and needles or tingling in the leg and or foot), so these lying twists will be beneficial to alleviate 'piriformis syndrome'. Ask the teacher for more piriformis stretch poses, if you think this is relevant to you.

Variation PROGRESSIVE 12iii

✓ Strengthens the abdominal obliques, the waist and back muscles.
✓ Stretches and mobilises the vertebral joints throughout the whole spine.
✓ Emphasizes the twist effects higher up the spine than previous versions.

All Variations

✓   Relieves tension in the musculature of the trunk.

✓   Creates space for, stimulates and brings health to the organs of the trunk.

✓   Stimulates or calms (balances) the nervous system.

✓   Increases energy levels and enthusiasm for life.

✓   Lifts fatigue and depression.

✓   See other benefits at CORE Lying Twists.

Related Yoga Poses

Parivrtta Trikonasana, Parivrtta Parsvakonasana, Garudasana, Ardha Matsyendrasana, Marichyasana III, Bharadvajasana.

RECLINED COBBLER POSE
– *Supta Baddha Konasana*
Refs.: CORE No. 13 PROGRESSIVE No. 13

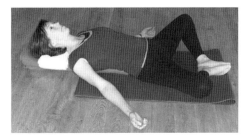

How to Perform the Pose

Sit on the floor, with a pillow behind you and 6 inches away, with your knees bent. Lower yourself down onto your elbows and then lie the back down onto the lengthwise pillow, placing a book/block or firm cushion on the top of the end of the pillow under your head and neck. Bring your feet in close to the body and on an exhalation allow your knees to relax out to the sides, bringing the soles of the feet together. Support the thighs with further cushions, if necessary, for comfort (or have a belt from knee to knee). Take the arms out by the sides with palms up. Stay for 1–3 minutes, if comfortable. To exit the pose, use your hands to lift the knees up.

After the pose: Place the feet well apart and allow the knees to drop inwards to touch each other and rest for a few moments, observing the counterbalancing broadness at the back of the pelvis.

Observations

▦   The pillow should be long enough to support the head too. If not, place several books/blocks, folded blankets or cushions under the head in order that the forehead is higher than the chin.

- The pillow supports from approximately the waist upwards, but the positioning should be very comfortable (some prefer the support an inch or two higher or lower than the waist).
- Take the skin and muscles at the back of the waist and the tailbone downwards towards the feet to lessen the lumbar curve.
- Using the hands, take the skin and muscles of the back of the pelvis from the centre to the sides; imagine a broad saucer at the back of the pelvis and the legs relaxing outwards only from the hip joints.
- Make sure the knees are level; if the feet are not in the centre, then one knee will appear higher and the back will not feel comfortable.
- If the feet are in the centre and one knee is still higher, then take support of cushions and/or blocks under both outer thighs until the knees are level.
- Take the arms lower down, if the arms or hands become uncomfortable in any way (e.g. if tingling occurs in the fingers).
- **This is a wonderful pose, so do make sure the props are correct in order to be able to remain comfortable.**

Variations

- Take a belt in a medium-sized loop and place it across the outer knees (this lessens the downward movement of the knees) for absolute comfort and relaxation in the groins, back and knees.
- Fold the arms up and over the head for more length and 'vertical' stretch.
- Bring the hands onto the abdomen for more abdominal relaxation and/or to encourage a deeper breath.
- Lie flat on the floor with no pillow.
- Have the feet near a wall or piece of furniture, to prevent the feet slipping away.
- Tuck rolled blankets or firm cushions under the outer hips on both sides to lessen groin stretch or to prevent pain at outer hips or shaking of the legs.
- For knee comfort, support the knees with firm supports or use a looped belt from knee to knee (belt on from outside, i.e. do not thread feet through belt).
- Imagine a clock-face at the back of the pelvis and take the time to relax around all the numbers of the clock (from 12 at the tailbone and around via the waist); lastly relax and sink the centre of the clock.

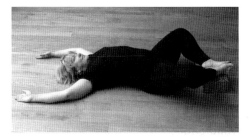

RECLINED COBBLER POSE (WITH FEET ON SUPPORT) – *Supta Baddha Konasana*

■ Lie flat on the floor with no pillow, but put the feet up on a few books/blocks for support (especially for a more comfortable low back/waist area, if one has a tendency to a sway back= an overly curved lumbar spine).

■ Whilst sitting to prepare, take a large loop of belt over the head and down to the back of the pelvis. Open the knees to the sides, take the belt inside the thighs and place the toes and feet into the belt. Tighten the belt to a comfortable tightness, ensuring that the buckle does not press into the skin and that the belt remains at the back of the sacrum and does not ride up around the waist. (Keeps the feet in, encourages lumbar length, supports the tendons of the groins, encourages inner thigh length and relaxation, binds the sacroiliac joints, makes the pose more intense, gives the body something to relax into.) Ask your teacher for a demonstration.

■ Try crossing the legs instead (Supta Sukkhasana) with a belt from knee to knee; equal time in both leg crosses.

■ Lie along the pillow as in the basic pose, but instead of a book/block for the head, take a blanket fanned to be approximately 3–4 feet long, approximately 4 inches wide and approximately 1–3 inches thick and place one end under the lower back ribs with the top end folded over double for extra height for the head. This will give a 3 step look rather than a 2 step look.

Benefits

✓ Stretches the groins and inner thigh muscles.

✓ Brings mobility to the hip-joints, allowing less overuse of the lower back, e.g. when getting out of a car or off a bike.

✓ Decreases disc bulges and can help to heal herniated discs.

✓ Opens the front of the spine and the front of the body.

✓ Space is created within the pelvic, abdominal and thoracic cavities.

✓ Releases tension within the pelvic and shoulder girdles.

- ✓ Encourages health in the organs of the pelvis (especially reproductive organs and bladder), abdomen (especially bowel and stomach) and the chest (lungs and heart).
- ✓ Encourages blood-flow to, and space and ease to, the heart.
- ✓ Stretches and relaxes the abdominals.
- ✓ Relaxes and encourages efficient use of the diaphragm.
- ✓ Stretches the intercostal muscles of the front and side ribs, allowing greater freedom for the breath.
- ✓ The antidote to stress for the body and the mind.
- ✓ May boost the immune system.
- ✓ Emotional stability and tranquillity is gained.
- ✓ Can lower the blood pressure.
- ✓ Lessens or prevents prostate problem symptoms.
- ✓ Can lessen or prevent menopausal/menstrual symptoms.
- ✓ Energising for body and mind.
- ✓ Lifts depression and gives feeling of hope and happiness.
- ✓ Lessens anxiety.
- ✓ Reduces fatigue and enlivens.
- ✓ Very useful therapeutic pose for most ailments, physical, physiological, emotional or mental.

Related Yoga Poses
Baddha Konasana, Supta Sukkhasana.

DOUBLE LEG LOCK – Supta Pavanamuktasana
Refs.: CORE No. 14 PROGRESSIVE No. 14

What To Do If… No. 3g

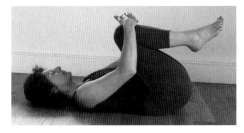

How to Perform the Pose
Lie on your back and on an exhalation bring your knees in towards your chest. Hold the knees with your arms, by interlocking your fingers past your shins. Have a book/block under your head, if necessary, to keep your chin at the same height as your forehead (never above that height). Remain still and breathe steadily.

– JELLY WOBBLE
Ref.: CORE No. 14i

How to Perform the Pose
Keeping your body relaxed, jiggle your legs in and out (an inch or two) in a fairly minimal and quick way so that your whole body relaxes and wobbles. Up to 60 seconds.

Observations
- Observe how the skin, flesh, muscles and bones seem to move like separate layers as you relax and jiggle more.
- Keep the movement small and relaxed; no jerks.
- Notice how the wobble goes all the way up to the head.
- Relax the facial muscles.
- Relax the back muscles.

– SPINAL ROCK
Refs.: CORE No. 14ii PROGRESSIVE No. 14ii

How to Perform the Pose
Slowly and comfortably rock from side to side, observing your back's contact with the floor and allowing your back to feel massaged by the floor. Up to 60 seconds. Then hold still for up to 60 seconds.

Observations
- Observe the spine and back muscles.
- Observe the gravitational effects as different parts are leaned into.
- Observe how some parts of the back are more tender or bony than others, but how the more often this is done, the more comfort and evenness is felt.
- If the bones of the middle of the back feel they are getting bruised, take the knees a little further away (extra blanket or double mat padding can be used under the body).
- If the back of the pelvis feels too tender, try bringing the knees a little closer in.

- Should there be restriction or tenderness at the front of the groins when bringing the knees in: ease the knees away and relax the muscles and tendons at the front hips (less cordlike tension) and bring the knees in slowly on the exhalation with relaxation. It is not necessary to bring the knees in to the maximum.
- Imagine the direction of the front of the legs to be up the shins to the knees and on to the front of the hips; flex the ankles to feel these directions more clearly.
- Keep the arms, shoulders and face relaxed.

Variations
- This is best done on a firm floor, but if very tender, perform with more softness underneath, e.g. a thicker carpet, or fold up a blanket with even layers.
- Ease the knees in with the exhalations and ease the knees away with the inhalations.
- Go very slowly so that it feels more like a lean to one side and a hold.
- Move faster to build up warmth.
- Go as far to the side as is possible, to lean onto the side hips and the back of the shoulders.
- Take the head the opposite way to the knees so that a slight twisting element is added or alternatively keep a tight relationship of the knees to the chest to prevent any twist and to build up more abdominal strength.
- Have the knees and feet a little apart for more broadness to the back body.

CIRCLE THE KNEES – *Supta Pavanamuktasana*
Ref.: PROGRESSIVE No. 14i

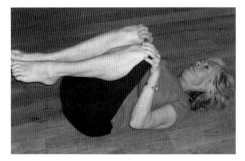

How to Perform the Pose
Placing your hands on your kneecaps and keeping your knees together, slowly circle both knees around one way twice and then back around the other way twice. Repeat up to 5 times. Hold your knees into your chest and remain still for 30 seconds.

Observations

▨ Notice how the back feels and aim to encourage more symmetry afterwards.

▨ Observe how one way may feel perfect and the other way not so useful.

▨ Move slowly and steadily.

Benefits

✓ Massages the back.

✓ Stimulates acupressure points for pain relief.

✓ Mobilises the joints of the back.

✓ Strengthens the abdominal and side waist muscles.

✓ Brings awareness of tender areas, thereby allowing one to relax these areas on the exhalations.

✓ Comfort for the back.

✓ Very gentle stretching of the facet joint capsules.

✓ Opening up and massaging of the facet joint area for their health.

✓ Gentle stretching of the lower back muscles.

✓ Reduces any inflammatory conditions (joint capsules, muscles, etc.) for long-term health.

✓ Reduces wind and constipation.

✓ The first 'forward bend' action after a herniated disc, encouraging healthy healing of the disc wall.

✓ Comforting and secure pose.

✓ Learn to be still in a comfortable position.

✓ Lessens lumbar lordosis (inward curve/sway back).

✓ Prepares the body for lying flat.

✓ Brings the body back to compact symmetry.

Related Yoga Poses

Adho Mukha Virasana, Malasana.

RELAXATION – *Savasana*
Refs.: CORE No. 15 PROGRESSIVE No. 15

What To Do If... No. 2b

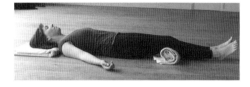

How to Perform the Pose
Sit on the floor with your knees bent and soles of feet on the floor and your hands behind you. Place a pillow or rolled blanket under where your knees are. Gently lower your back down onto the floor, placing a book or folded blanket under your neck and head in order that your forehead is level with, or slightly higher than, your chin. Keep the back of your neck long. Tilt the pelvis by taking the tailbone down and use your hands to spread the buttock flesh out to the sides. Gently close your eyes. With your hands on the abdomen to observe that the pelvis and abdomen do not get disturbed, take your legs out along the floor one at a time, placing a rolled blanket or pillow under your knees. You may prefer to have the legs bent and up on a chair-seat, sofa or bed as in CORE 15 (photograph below).

RELAXATION WITH LEGS ON CHAIR-SEAT – *Savasana*
Ref.: What To Do If... No. 2a CORE 15 PROGRESSIVE 15

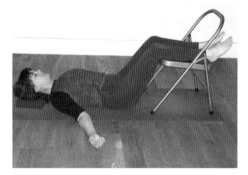

You may also progress to taking your legs completely straight along the floor, provided this is absolutely comfortable. Close the eyes and stay for 5–20 minutes, making some of the following observations to keep the mind steady and focused. To exit the pose, see below at the end of observations.

Observations
- Listen to the '*Yoga For Healthy Lower Backs* Relaxations CD' often; begin with Track 1, but later choose the track that suits you best or use different tracks for variety.
- Allow the legs to relax from the feet to the hip joints.
- Sink the navel on the exhalations.

- Encourage a spreading of the lower side ribs on the inhalations.
- Relax the front of the ribs.
- Spread the collarbones from the centre to the sides to allow the shoulders to relax down and out to the right and left.
- Relax the sides of the trunk from the side hips to the side armpits.
- Relax the back of the shoulders and allow them to sink into the floor, releasing tension there on each exhalation.
- Relax the shoulder blades and the upper back.
- Relax the back of the waist, encouraging the relaxation to move from the centre to the sides of the waist.
- Relax the lower back.
- Relax the back of the pelvis.
- Feel the spine lengthen within the relaxed trunk from tailbone to the head.
- Relax the fingers and the hands.
- Relax the arms from the fingertips to the shoulders.
- Have a feeling of spreading as the muscles relax.
- Allow the bones to sink.
- Relax the sides of the neck to behind the ears.
- Relax the back of the neck from between the shoulder blades to the base of the skull.
- Relax the back of the head and relax the top of the head.
- Relax the forehead skin from the hairline down to the eyes.
- Soften the eyelids.
- Soften the skin of the cheeks and allow the cheekbones to sink.
- Soften the skin of the lips.
- Relax the jaw from the ears to the chin and have space between the lower and upper teeth.
- Allow the tongue to rest away from the roof of the mouth behind the lower teeth and to have a feeling of shrinking as it relaxes.
- Sink the eyes into their sockets and turn them down towards the centre of the chest.
- Allow the energy of the brain to move down towards the chest.
- Breathe softly, smoothly and steadily.
- Stay as long as feels comfortable and aim to keep the mind in check by clearing it with your steady exhalations.
- Note the joy, comfort and positivity of the moment and allow this to spread throughout your day.

- Note your physical and mental state and allow that to become more a part of yourself.
- **To exit the pose**: take a few steady deep breaths to re-energise your body and your mind. Gently move your fingers and then rest your hands on your abdomen. Gently move your toes and feet and slowly bend one leg at a time to place your feet on the floor with your knees bent. On an exhalation and without twisting, gently roll yourself completely onto your right side and, making sure your head is supported on something, rest for a few breaths. On another exhalation, roll onto your back again. On another exhalation, roll over onto your left side and rest for a few more breaths. When you feel ready to come up, do not use your back muscles, but keep your head and chest facing towards the floor, use your arms to bring you up to a sitting position on an exhalation. Inhale well once you are sitting upright. Slowly come up off the floor, making the effort on the exhalation, without rushing, and using a chair or piece of furniture for support if necessary. Inhale once upright and breathe normally.
- Enjoy the moment.

Variations

- Lie along a lengthwise pillow as in Reclined Cobbler Pose CORE 13 (for health of the discs and comfort of the sacroiliac joints) and have the legs straight (for space for the discs) or bent (for the relaxation of the back muscles) **See photograph for Pranayama (Breathing Awareness).**
- Lie prone (tummy down) with a pillow under the abdomen and chest (for herniated or bulging discs, perform 3 x a day for 5–10 mins.) **See PRONE LYING photograph under Pose of Child** CORE No. 9i.
- Aim to often emulate some of the mental and physical responses and effects in different positions, e.g. whilst sat in a chair, whilst stuck at a red traffic light or whilst having a difficult phone conversation.

Benefits

- ✓ Relieves pain.
- ✓ Relaxes the physical body.
- ✓ Calms the physiological systems of the body.
- ✓ Brings clarity to the mind.
- ✓ Brings stability and equilibrium to the emotions.
- ✓ Enhances energy levels.
- ✓ Brings equanimity in facing life's challenges.

✓   Brings a feeling of tranquility.

✓   Reduces stress.

✓   Relieves anxiety.

✓   Lifts depression (especially if done after some active yoga and along a lengthwise pillow – do the relaxation with the eyes softly open if that feels better).

✓   Boosts the immune system.

✓   Allows homeostasis of the body, equilibrium and balance of all the systems of the body: endocrine; respiratory; cardiovascular; nervous; digestive; eliminatory; reproductive; lymph; etc.

✓   Creates a positive mood.

✓   Puts life in perspective.

✓   Increases productivity.

✓   Allows the benefits of any previous yoga to manifest within the body for long-term health and positive change.

✓   WONDER POSE – one of the best tools you will ever have! So practise and get better at it.

BREATHING AWARENESS – *Pranayama* (Simplified)

Refs.: CORE No. 15 PROGRESSIVE No. 15

What To Do If... No. 2c

(Often Best With Legs On Chair-Seat)

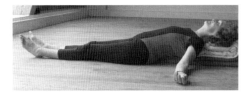

How to Perform the Pose

Lie comfortably on your back in Savasana with your eyes closed (photo above shows blanket support and you could lie your trunk along a pillow to open the chest well plus have a book/block on top of that for extra head support). It is not necessary to do this breathing awareness practice every time, so just do some of it, when you feel you want to. It is good to use the '*Yoga for Healthy Lower Backs* Relaxations CD' Track 3 for this. Never rush or strain. You may spend from 1–20 minutes doing some or all of these gentle basic yoga breathing exercises.

Observations

- Observe the breath as it is.
- Observe the breath within the pelvic and abdominal areas and encourage the breath to move there.
- Observe the breath within the ribcage and encourage the breath to move in the front, side and back ribs. The ribs should lift and separate. The lower floating ribs spread to the sides and the back ribs are felt on the floor.
- Observe the breath within the top chest and encourage the collarbones to lift up towards the face.
- Keep the eyes looking down towards the chest throughout.
- Observe the inhalation of the breath moving upwards from deep down in the pelvis, into the chest and on up to the top chest.

– SINKING OF THE NAVEL ON THE EXHALATIONS

- Observe the sinking of the navel as you exhale.
- Observe how this allows more space for the inhalations.

– INTERRUPTED EXHALATIONS (*Viloma Pranayama*)

▧ Complete a full inhalation to prepare.
▧ Gently start to breathe out a little and hold, then breathe out a little more and hold, breathe out a little more and so on until the exhalation is complete. Use timings that seem comfortable to you – do not be dictated to by your mind or the timings in other yoga books. Breathe normally for a few breaths. Then repeat one more breath in the same way. Breathe normally for several 'recovery and observational' breaths.

– INTERRUPTED INHALATIONS (*Viloma Pranayama*)

▧ **Do not do this if you tend towards high blood pressure**.
▧ Complete a full exhalation to prepare.
▧ Gently start to breathe in a little and hold, then breathe in a little more and hold, breathe in a little more and so on until the inhalation is complete. **Use timings that seem comfortable to you** – do not be dictated to by your mind or other yoga books. Breathe normally for a few breaths. Then repeat one more breath in the same way. Breathe normally for several 'recovery and observational' breaths.

– SAVASANA AFTER *Pranayama*

(Always rest well after pranayama)
Relax and allow the breath to be subtle, smooth, steady and silky for a while. When you want to finish, first relax for a minute or two. Just relax, without any thoughts of the breath. Take your time to come up in the usual way, by rolling to the right, then to the left, etc.

Benefits
✓ Focusing on the breath can prevent the chatter of the mind; encouraging the mind to be calm will aid relaxation.
✓ Exhalations reduce anxiety.
✓ Exhalations calm the mind and steady the emotions.
✓ Exhalations lower the blood pressure.
✓ Inhalations energise.

✓ Inhalations inspire.

✓ Inhalations lift the mood.

✓ Balance of those two necessary parts of human potential: inward and outward; reaching outwards and going inside; being outgoing/sociable and being introspective/contemplative; loving the world and everything in it and loving all aspects of yourself.

✓ The breath can reduce tension from the inside out, where sometimes exterior physical exercises/stretching are not so effective.

✓ This involves prana – the lifeforce energy. Humans need to breathe for life!

✓ Greater efficiency of the breath.

✓ Health for the lungs.

✓ Health, exhilaration and invigoration for the mind.

✓ Mental clarity.

✓ Decisiveness.

✓ **Appreciation for life as it is**.

✓ Being in the **present** moment as the only **true** moment.

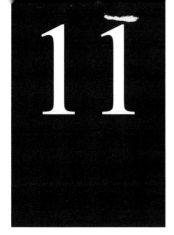

11 Twelve Weekly Class Themes

These 12 weekly class themes represent many of the concepts and ideas that are covered during a 12-class *Yoga for Healthy Lower Backs* course. The following represent some of the ideas followed for each class theme.

Themes

1. **Introduction to Yoga**
    Relaxation (*sukha*)– Soften and Pacify – "Let Go and Relax"

2. **Steadiness of Body, Breath, Mind** – (*sthita/dharana*) – "Steady and Still – Quiet Mind"

3. **Posture + Symmetry** – *(asana)* – Comfortable, Confident and Efficient within Body – "How to Stand, Sit and Lie Comfortably"

4. **Awareness** – (*svadhyaya/sarira prajna*) self-observation – "You have a Body all the time, NOT just when it aches"

5. **Mobility** – movement (*karmayoga*) – health to the joints – "Get out the oil-can!"

6. **Height, Space, Lift** – Defy Gravity (*rajas/akash*) – "Lift Off and Grow Tall"

7. **'Intelligence' and Life** – (*prana prajna*) Body wants to be Healthy and Comfortable – Potential for Health – The Soul wants to allow happiness to shine out – "Your Cells are Full of Life"

8. Stretch – Space for Joints – Healthy Muscles – Increased Circulation – Antidote to Stress (*moksa*) – "Don't Turn into Tanned Leather – Stretch and Release"

9. Strengthen – Body, Mind and Belief in Yoga (*sthira*) – "Stronger in Body and Mind"

10. Added Benefits – (*saucha*/*sarva*) e.g. less anxious, enhanced immune function, fewer headaches, lower blood pressure – not Just Health for Low Back, but also organs and systems, e.g. endocrine, nervous, digestive, respiratory, excretory, cardiovascular, senses – "Feeling 'Wholistically' Healthy"

11. Positivity – Notice Improvements, Acknowledge Path to Comfort, Health and Happiness – (*ananda*) – "Power of Intention"

12. Long-term – Reinforce Reasons Why we Continue to do Yoga (*tapas/ sadhana*), e.g. facets joints need movement; muscles need to be use;, tissues need to know they are needed; circulation is aided by movement and muscle use; discs need movement and horizontal rest for health; when the mind is at ease so is the body – possible to slip gracefully and effortlessly into mature age without disability – yogis are the example e.g. Yogacharya Sri B.K.S. Iyengar – Opportunities for Further Yoga Classes or How to Continue to Practice at Home – "Keep Up Your Yoga"

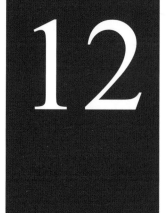

12 Anatomy of the Back

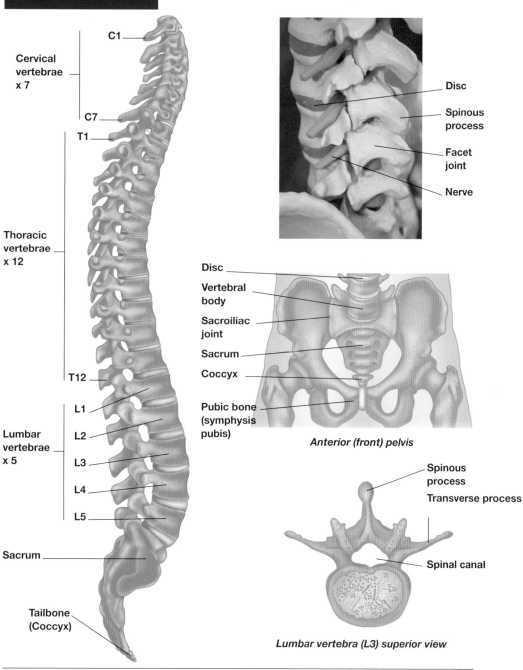

Cervical vertebrae x 7

C1

C7

T1

Disc

Spinous process

Facet joint

Nerve

Thoracic vertebrae x 12

Disc

Vertebral body

Sacroiliac joint

Sacrum

Coccyx

Pubic bone (symphysis pubis)

T12

L1

L2

Lumbar vertebrae x 5

L3

L4

L5

Anterior (front) pelvis

Spinous process

Transverse process

Spinal canal

Sacrum

Tailbone (Coccyx)

Lumbar vertebra (L3) superior view

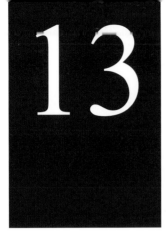

Warning Signs

If you have severe pain which gets worse over several weeks instead of better, or which never goes away, or if you are unwell with back pain, you should see your doctor.

Here are a few symptoms, which are all very rare, but if you do have back pain and suddenly develop any of these you should see a doctor straight away. These are listed by Professor Kim Burton et al in the *Back Book*.

- Difficulty passing or controlling urine

- Numbness around your back passage, genitals or inner thighs

- Loss of control and feeling from your back passage

- Numbness, pins and needles or weakness <u>in both legs</u>

- Unsteadiness on your feet

If You Visit Your GP

Please let your yoga teacher know if you have felt the need to visit your GP or other therapist about your back.

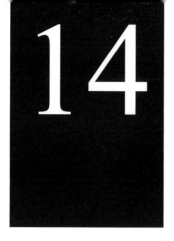

14 National Yoga Organisations

The British Wheel of Yoga (BWY)

25 Jermyn Street, Sleaford, Lincs, NG34 7RU   01529 306851

office@bwy.org.uk   *www.bwy.org.uk*

The British Wheel of Yoga is the Sport England recognized governing body for yoga. BWY is also the largest yoga organisation in the UK with over 3,750 qualified teachers. The website will help you to find teachers in your locality through either an online search or you could ring your county representative who will have a complete list of qualified British Wheel of Yoga teachers. They have been supportive of this research trial.

Iyengar Yoga Association of the United Kingdom, IYA (UK)

admin@iyengaryoga.org.uk   *www.iyengaryoga.org.uk*

Iyengar Yoga is one of the most widely-practised methods of yoga in the UK and indeed worldwide. As well as giving information about Iyengar Yoga and providing an easy search for teachers in particular areas of the country, this website will also guide people to local Iyengar Yoga Centres and Institutes via links to their websites.

The Iyengar Yoga Association (UK) has been supportive of this trial and this yoga programme from the outset and believe in its value, and they and the authors would like to thank respected Yogacharya Sri B.K.S. Iyengar for all the knowledge that he has shared. The Ramamani Iyengar Memorial Yoga Institute in Pune, India wishes it to be known that this manual does not aim to represent the format that they would use within their highly-respected, specialist Medical Classes in Pune. This manual has been designed for newcomers to yoga for introductory-type classes with a focus on the health of the lower back.

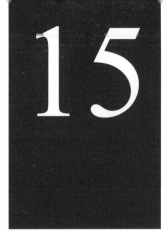

15 Four Day Training Course

Yoga teachers qualified to teach the *Yoga for Healthy Lower Backs* yoga programme, as contained within this manual, will have completed a four-day training course, along with home study, mentor support and a trainee course.

Four Day 12-Week Training Course

- Open to qualified yoga teachers with considerable post-qualification experience of yoga teaching
- Intensive course over two weekends, with several months' break between weekends for consolidation of learning
- Extensive home yoga practice and study reading is required
- Backed by email and other tutorial/mentoring assistance during the trainee teaching of the first 12-week course
- Yoga teachers who satisfactorily complete the training course will be listed on the www.yogaforbacks.co.uk site as qualified teachers

Details of training opportunities will be regularly updated on the *www.yogaforbacks.co.uk* website.

Pain

10 million people in the UK are affected by arthritis and related conditions.

Relief

Research is our best hope of a future free from the pain caused by arthritis.

Arthritis Research UK
Providing answers today and tomorrow

Arthritis Research UK is **the** charity leading the fight against arthritis. Our aim is to take the pain away for millions of sufferers of all forms of arthritis and help them remain active throughout their lives.

We do this by funding high quality research, providing information so that people can make informed decisions about their treatments and lifestyle and campaigning to improve the quality of life for sufferers.

If you would like more information, call us on **0870 850 5000** or visit **www.arthritisresearchuk.org**

Registered Charity England and Wales no. 207711, Scotland no. SC041156

Alison Trewhela

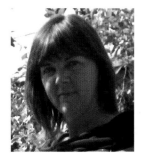 Alison Trewhela (Iyengar Yoga certificated; SBRCP-Yoga, Senior Practitioner, Institute of Complementary and Natural Medicine) has taught yoga regularly since 1983, when she began teaching in The Bahamas. She teaches mainly in Cornwall (but also in Switzerland), including some small group and individual therapeutic yoga, and teaches yoga workshops throughout the UK. Since the inception of the Peninsula Medical School in Cornwall, she has led medical students in studies into yoga's therapeutic physical, mental and spiritual benefits.

In 1992-1993, Alison qualified in The Yoga Biomedical Trust's specialist yoga teachers' course for Lower Back Pain. With this interest in back pain diagnostics and treatment along with her Iyengar Yoga knowledge, she soon designed and set up 7-week Better Back Courses for newcomers to yoga with low back pain and, whilst continually updating and improving them, received referrals from GPs, hospital pain clinics, physiotherapists, acupuncturists, osteopaths and others.

Over the years, Alison has contributed to the Iyengar Yoga community by acting as Chair of the SW Iyengar Yoga Institute, Secretary for LOYA as it merged with the BKSIYTA to become IYA (UK), and has played major parts in helping to run national conventions. Alison is indebted to all her teachers and students and is eternally grateful for all the knowledge and wisdom that has been graciously passed down from the Iyengar family in Pune. She has gained inspiration by completing Iyengar Yoga Therapy workshops with Stephanie Quirk and classes with Richard Agar Ward and Ali Dashti.

Alison designed this book's yoga programme and enjoyed working with Anna Semlyen on the University of York's yoga trial team, 2005-2011, including manual-writing, taking photos and recording the Relaxations CD. She trains teachers in the full *Yoga for Healthy Lower Backs* programme.
www.yogatrewhela.co.uk   alan@trewhela5090.freeserve.co.uk.

Anna Semlyen

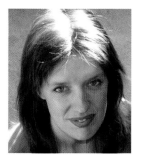Anna Semlyen, (BA MA Philosophy, Politics, Economics (Oxon), MSc Health Economics (York), British Wheel of Yoga (BWY) Dip, Ayurveda Foundations, Reiki 2) has taught yoga since 1996. Her business is called Yoga in York. Anna learnt yoga for lower back care with Alison Trewhela and at BWY In Service Training courses, plus experience of her own back care classes. Anna is Specialist Advisor to the BWY on Yoga and Healthy Backs and also Research on Therapeutic Yoga. Anna worked for the NHS 1992-3 and then as a Health Economics Research Fellow at The University of York 1993-1998 before becoming a full-time yoga teacher.

She contributed to yoga research 2005-2011. From 2007 preparation of the *Yoga for Healthy Lower Backs* manuals for students and teachers and a Relaxations CD (collaborative projects with Alison) for the University of York's trial were funded by Arthritis Research UK.

Anna teaches many weekly general and therapeutic yoga classes, private lessons and also trains yoga teachers. She has taught at BWY National Congress and is a BWY In Service Training Tutor on the *Yoga for Healthy Lower Backs* programme, plus Yoga and Ayurvedic Dosha (constitutions), Mental Health and Concentration.

This is her sixth book. She has had research papers published and many articles in yoga magazines. She has recorded two relaxation CDs. She is grateful for opportunities to learn, teach and research yoga and for everyone who has made this possible.

www.yogainyork.co.uk anna@yogainyork.co.uk

Both authors can also be contacted via the website *www.yogaforbacks.co.uk.*

Authors' Vision

The authors have a vision that in the future these scientifically-proven *Yoga for Healthy Lower Backs* courses will be offered under the UK NHS and private health insurance schemes and, maybe similarly, in other countries too.

We would be grateful if you feel you could help us with that aim by informing GPs, PCTs (Primary Health Care Trusts), health promotion departments, large employers, hospitals, health insurance providers, yoga teachers, yoga students and the general public with chronic low back pain about this research, these courses and this book. Info on www.yogaforbacks.co.uk.

Thank you.